NURSING CARE OF THE LABOR PATIENT

edition 2

NURSING CARE OF THE LABOR PATIENT
edition 2

**JANET SWANSON MALINOWSKI,
R.N., M.S.N.**
ASSOCIATE PROFESSOR OF NURSING
MERCY COLLEGE OF DETROIT
DETROIT, MICHIGAN

F.A. DAVIS COMPANY ● PHILADELPHIA

Library of Congress Cataloging in Publication Data
Main entry under title:

Nursing care of the labor patient.

  Includes bibliographies and index.
  1. Obstetrical nursing. 2. Labor (Obstetrics)
I. Malinowski, Janet S. [DNLM: 1. Obstetrical nursing
—Programmed texts. WY 18 M251n]
RG951.N87 1983   618.4'024613   82-22081
ISBN 0-8036-5802-8

PREFACE

The nature and approach of this book's second edition remain the same as the first. The book presents material essential for nursing practice in the area of labor and delivery. It is written in a clear, concise, and organized way, using a programmed approach. The objectives and self-test questions in each chapter facilitate the reader's understanding of the topic. The book addresses all educational levels of basic nursing. It can serve as an introduction to, a reference for, or a review of nursing care of the labor patient.

This edition is purposefully more in-depth than the first. The extensive use of electronic monitoring, the involvement of fathers (or their substitutes), the testing of fetal response, and alternatives to traditional childbirth methods are additions to the book that reflect the current trends in these areas. These additions and numerous others update the book and should make it more valuable for the student nurse as well as the graduate nurse, who finds nursing knowledge and technology to be ever changing.

Janet S. Malinowski

CONTRIBUTORS

CAROLYN PEDIGO DELOACH, R.N., M.S.N.
Associate Professor of Nursing
Eastern Michigan University
Ypsilanti, Michigan

JOYCE BAGROWSKI MCCABE, R.N., M.S.N.
Clinical Nurse Specialist in Perinatology
Oakwood Hospital
Dearborn, Michigan
Formerly, Assistant Professor of Nursing
Mercy College of Detroit
Detroit, Michigan

PATRICIA DYER WILLIAMS, R.N., B.S.N.
Head Nurse, Antepartum-Postpartum Unit
Women's Hospital, The University of Michigan Hospitals;
Formerly, Childbirth Educator in Lamaze Method; and
Lecturer in Nursing
The University of Michigan
Ann Arbor, Michigan

DIRECTIONS TO THE READER

As you start each chapter of this book, carefully read the stated OBJEC-TIVES. They tell you what you should gain from your reading.

Periodically, throughout each chapter, REVIEW QUESTIONS will be asked. They cover the material immediately preceding them. Space is provided so that you can write down your answers. Your written responses help you remember the most important content. They also serve as an immediate reward if your answers are correct.

In order to reinforce your correct answers and to dispel any incorrect ones, ANSWERS are immediately provided. They are written in such a way that review of the content could be done just by reading the answers. This is not recommended for the first reading but might be an appropriate method when a quick review is desirable—for example, before an exam in school or State Boards.

At the end of each chapter is a POST-TEST. This is a cumulative evaluation of your understanding of the content addressed in the chapter's objectives. Again, there is space for your answers and immediate feedback from the printed answers.

This programmed approach should enhance your understanding and retention of the book's content.

Janet S. Malinowski

CONTENTS

CHAPTER 1

AN OVERVIEW OF NURSING CARE DURING LABOR AND DELIVERY

Carolyn Pedigo DeLoach

Labor generally begins at 38 to 42 weeks gestation, when the fetus is mature enough to cope with extrauterine conditions, but not so large that mechanical difficulties result during labor and delivery. Even though the mother may have experienced the normal developmental stages of pregnancy, labor and delivery can be an acute developmental and situational crisis for her. With skillful intervention by the health care team the negative impact of the experience can be decreased, and the birth experience can be positive. It can even foster stronger relationships among all family members.

This chapter is divided into two parts. The first part, the labor and delivery process, focuses on essential terminology that is fundamental to nursing care; the second part focuses on nursing care during the labor and delivery process. Emphasis is placed on assessing labor progress. Some methods of facilitating maternal coping behaviors are given.

OBJECTIVES

Upon completion of this chapter, the reader will be able to:

1. Briefly explain the commonly accepted theories of the cause of labor.
2. Explain the significance of the following for a normal course of labor and delivery:

continued on next page

      a. premonitory signs of labor
      b. rupture of membranes
      c. physiologic/psychologic aspects of the four stages of labor
      d. fetal lie and attitude, presentation, position, and station
      e. mechanisms of labor.
3.   Distinguish between false labor and true labor.
4.   Describe at least five physiologic/psychologic changes that the nurse should recognize as significant signs of progress in labor.
5.   Identify nursing measures that:
      a. assess maternal/fetal well-being
      b. provide comfort during labor
      c. promote parent-newborn attachment.
6.   Describe nursing responsibilities related to:
      a. the four stages of labor
      b. the unexpected, unattended birth
      c. immediate care of the newborn.

THE LABOR AND DELIVERY PROCESS

Theories of Labor

There are several scientific explanations for the onset of labor. The following theories are most widely accepted.

PROGESTERONE DEPRIVATION THEORY. Throughout pregnancy there is a balance between estrogen and progesterone. Progesterone, produced by the placenta, is crucial to the maintenance of the pregnancy, because it inhibits uterine muscular activity. As production of progesterone decreases near term, uterine contraction activity increases, initiating labor. Since there is no documented evidence of decreased progesterone levels prior to labor, progesterone may have only an indirect effect upon the onset of labor.

OXYTOCIN STIMULATION THEORY. Oxytocin, secreted by the anterior pituitary gland, stimulates the uterine muscles to contract. The uterus becomes increasingly sensitive to oxytocin prior to and during labor. It is theorized that oxytocin initiates labor and causes progressive labor contractions.

UTERINE STRETCH THEORY. The overdistended uterus exerts pressure on nerve endings, theoretically causing increased irritability of the uterus with subsequent labor contractions. This may partially explain why the presence of multiple gestation, a large fetus, or excessive amniotic fluid (hydramnios/polyhydramnios) may result in premature onset of labor.

PLACENTAL DEGENERATION THEORY. Thrombi at the placental site begin to form between 33 to 36 weeks gestation. This results in decreased circulation and oxygenation, which causes placental degeneration (aging). This may trigger the onset of labor.

ESTROGEN STIMULATION THEORY. Estrogen causes an increased level of contractile proteins, hypertrophy (enlargement) of the uterine muscles, and formation of adenosine triphosphate (ATP), which is a source of energy for contractions. This combination is thought to promote the onset of labor.

FETAL MEMBRANE PHOSPHOLIPID-ARACHIDONIC ACID-PROSTAGLANDIN THEORY. It is theorized that the decrease in progesterone levels just before labor activates phospholipase A_2 which sets free arachidonic acid. This acid acts on prostaglandins (E_2, F_2) which stimulate contractions of uterine smooth muscles.

FETAL CORTISOL THEORY. The fetus may be an important contributor to the onset of labor. Research by Liggins[1] found that the onset of labor was delayed following removal of the adrenal cortex and pituitary glands in a fetal lamb. Conversely, initiation of premature labor in sheep has occurred as a result of administration of cortisol and ACTH.

Review Question

List and briefly explain four commonly accepted theories of the cause of labor onset.

a. _____

_____

_____

b. _____

_____

_____

c. _____

_____

_____

d. _____

_____

_____

Answer

Commonly accepted theories of the cause of labor are:

a. Progesterone Deprivation Theory. Progesterone inhibits uterine muscular activity. Uterine contraction activity increases as progesterone levels decrease toward term.

b. Oxytocin Stimulation Theory. Oxytocin stimulates uterine contractions.

c. Uterine Stretch Theory. Increased uterine irritability and subsequent contractions occur because of pressure on nerve endings from the overdistended uterus.

d. Placental Degeneration Theory. Degeneration (aging) caused by thrombi of the placenta initiates the onset of labor.

e. Estrogen Stimulation Theory. Estrogen causes increased levels of contractile proteins, myometrial hypertrophy, and formation of ATP to promote the onset of labor.

f. Fetal Membrane Phospholipid-Arachidonic Acid-Prostaglandin Theory. The interrelationship of actions of the above leads to increased levels of prostaglandins, which stimulate uterine smooth muscle contractions.

g. Fetal Cortisol Theory. Initiation of premature labor may occur with the administration of cortisol and ACTH. Delay of labor does occur with the removal of fetal adrenal cortex and pituitary gland in lambs.

Premonitory Signs of Labor

Although no one really knows the cause of labor, there are identifiable signs of approaching labor. They are called premonitory signs of labor.

ENGAGEMENT. This is the passage of the largest diameter of the fetal presenting part (usually the head) into the maternal pelvic inlet (brim). In the primigravida (first pregnancy) engagement may occur as early as two weeks prior to the onset of labor (see the section on Descent Patterns in Chapter 4). In the multigravida (second or more pregnancy), engagement usually does not occur until the onset of labor or later. Leg pain due to pressure on the sciatic nerve and urinary frequency due to uterine pressure on the bladder are common discomforts following engagement. Engagement should not be confused with the term lightening, which is the settling of the uterus and its contents into the pelvis.

UTERINE CONTRACTIONS. It is sometimes difficult to distinguish between Braxton-Hicks contractions *(false labor)* and contractions of true labor. Braxton-Hicks contractions, which occur throughout pregnancy, may become increasingly uncomfortable just prior to labor. They are irregular and do not increase in frequency, duration, or intensity. They do not cause cervical dilatation but may assist in ripening, i.e., softening, and thinning (effacement) of the cervix, and moving it forward (anterior) in the pelvis. The discomfort of Braxton-Hicks contractions can usually be lessened by walking. *True labor* contractions are regular and tend to increase in frequency, duration, and intensity as labor progresses. These contractions bring about progressive cervical changes and cause discomfort in the lower back and abdomen. Walking usually intensifies the contractions (see the section on Ambulation as a Labor Stimulant in Chapter 5).

CERVICAL CHANGES. True labor is diagnosed upon the occurrence of regular, rhythmic contractions which bring about progressive cervical dilatation (gradual opening of the cervix to 10 cm) and effacement (gradual thinning of the internal cervical os).

BLOODY SHOW. Prior to or during labor, the cervical mucous plug is expelled owing to pressure of the fetus and some cervical effacement. Cervical capillaries may rupture, causing blood to be mixed with cervical mucus. Bloody show is thick, mucousy, and pink or dark red. It must be differentiated from active vaginal bleeding which is thin, watery, and bright red. Active bleeding may indicate abnormalities of the placenta such as:

Placenta previa—a condition in which the placenta abnormally implants in the lower uterine segment. The previa is classified as *total,* if it completely covers the cervical os; *partial,* if it covers only a portion of the cervical os; or *marginal,* if it is implanted in close proximity to the cervical os. Placenta previa usually manifests with painless bleeding.

Abruptio placentae—a condition in which a normally implanted placenta separates from the uterine wall prior to delivery of the baby. The abruption may be *partial or total.* Maternal conditions that may increase the risk of abruption are maternal age greater than 30; more than five pregnancies; preeclampsia-eclampsia; renal or vascular disease; hydramnios; and multiple pregnancy. Abruptio placentae is most frequently associated with painful bleeding.

RUPTURE OF MEMBRANES (ROM). Spontaneous rupture of membranes (SROM) may occur before true labor starts or anytime during labor. Membranes may also be ruptured artificially (AROM). This procedure, called amniotomy, must be performed by a physician (see the section on Amniotomy as a Labor Stimulant in Chapter 5 for nursing interventions).

The amniotic fluid may gush or slowly trickle from the vagina. Normal fluid is clear or cloudy and colorless or pale yellow. The odor should not be strong or foul (indicating infection). The fluid may be cloudy due to the presence of vernix caseosa which is a white, cheeselike substance coating the fetal skin in utero. Meconium-stained (brown, black, or greenish color) amniotic fluid when the fetus presents head first indicates that at some point the fetus experienced distress causing anoxia. With anoxia the anal sphincter relaxes, resulting in expulsion of feces into the amniotic fluid. Meconium-stained amniotic fluid would be normal *only* when the fetus presents buttocks first. In this case, expulsion of feces is caused by cervical pressure on the fetal anus, not by anoxia.

The amount of amniotic fluid present in the term uterus is approximately 1000 ml. Some women fear that if the membranes rupture prior to the onset of labor, all the amniotic fluid will leave the uterine cavity and cause a dry birth. This is a fallacy. Not all the amniotic fluid leaves the uterine cavity at the time of ROM. Throughout the remainder of labor, amniotic fluid is expelled, especially during contractions and when the woman moves or changes position. Amniotic fluid continues to provide moisture and lubrication throughout labor.

Amniotic fluid in excess of 2000 to 3000 ml is classified as *hydramnios* or *polyhydramnios*. It is often associated with fetal malformations in which the fetus is unable to swallow and urinate normally in utero. Hydramnios is also associated with maternal disorders such as diabetes mellitus, Rh sensitization, and placental tumors.

Oligohydramnios is the term used to describe an extremely scant amount (less than 300 ml) of amniotic fluid that is very concentrated. The condition is rare and the cause is unknown, although it is associated with fetal renal disorders and postmaturity.

It is sometimes difficult to distinguish amniotic fluid from urine. At term, pressure from the enlarged uterus on the bladder may cause involuntary leakage of urine, especially when the pregnant women coughs or sneezes. Three tests are commonly used to establish the presence of amniotic fluid:

Nitrazine Test Tape. Amniotic fluid changes the color of nitrazine tape to blue-green, blue-gray, or dark blue—an alkaline reaction. Urine is acidic and does not change the color of the nitrazine tape. If a lubricant has been used for the vaginal exam prior to testing with nitrazine tape, false results may be obtained, that is, the tape will remain yellow, olive, or olive-green in color. This result without the interference of lubricant usually means probable intact membranes.

Staining of Fetal Fat Cells. Fetal fat cells are sloughed off into the amniotic fluid during the last weeks of a term pregnancy. The presence of fetal fat cells in the vaginal fluid is a positive way of identifying that the fluid is amniotic fluid. A small amount of amniotic fluid is placed on a slide. Nile blue sulfate added to the fluid causes fetal fat cells to stain orange.

Ferning of Cervical Mucus. During pregnancy, with the amniotic sac intact, cervical mucus is viscous and opaque. The mucus changes to a fernlike pattern of crystallization when mixed with amniotic fluid. Evidence of ferning of cervical mucus under a microscope indicates probable ROM.

OTHER PREMONITORY SIGNS OF LABOR. Additional subjective changes may occur just prior to the onset of labor. These changes may include *a sudden burst of energy.* Although the woman may want to use this energy for tasks she has neglected, she should refrain from doing so. This energy is needed for the work of labor. Other changes may include *increased backache, increased vaginal secretions, a sudden 2 to 3 pound weight loss* (from diuresis of retained fluid), and *loose stools or diarrhea.*

Review Questions

1. The passage of the largest diameter of the fetal presenting part into the maternal pelvic inlet is called _____ .

2. Differentiate between Braxton-Hicks contractions (false labor) and contractions that signal true labor by filling in the chart using the terms in column I.

Column I		Braxton-Hicks	True Labor
a.	**Discomfort**	a.	a.
b.	**Regularity**	b.	b.
c.	**Cervical dilatation**	c.	c.
d.	**Effect of walking**	d.	d.

3. During labor, cervical dilatation progresses to _____ cm.

4. Define effacement of the cervix. _____
_____
_____

5. Describe the differences in color and consistency between bloody show (normal) and active vaginal bleeding (abnormal).
_____
_____
_____

6. A condition in which the placenta abnormally implants in the lower uterine wall is called _____ _____ .

7. A condition in which a normally implanted placenta prematurely separates from the uterine wall is called _____
_____ .

8. The procedure by which the membranes are artificially ruptured is called _____ .

9. In each of the following, what does the presence of meconium-stained amniotic fluid indicate?
   a. If the fetus presents head first, meconium indicates:
   _____
   _____
   _____

   b. If the fetus presents buttocks first, meconium indicates:
   _____
   _____
   _____

10. An excessive amount of amniotic fluid associated with malformations in which the fetus is usually unable to swallow and urinate normally in utero is _____ .

11. Briefly describe three tests commonly used to document ROM.
   a. _____
   _____
   _____

   b. _____
   _____
   _____

   c. _____
   _____
   _____

Answers

1. *Engagement* is the passage of the largest diameter of the fetal presenting part into the maternal pelvic inlet.

2. The differences between Braxton-Hicks contractions (false labor) and contractions that signal true labor are:

Column I		Braxton-Hicks		True Labor
a.	Discomfort	a.	Occur throughout pregnancy; may become uncomfortable just prior to labor	a.	Increase in intensity and duration, causing discomfort in the lower back and abdomen
b.	Regularity	b.	Irregular	b.	Regular
c.	Cervical dilatation	c.	None	c.	Progressive cervical changes
d.	Effect of walking	d.	May decrease discomfort	d.	Intensifies contractions

3. Cervical dilatation progresses to *10 cm* during labor.

4. Effacement is the gradual thinning of the internal cervical os.

5. Bloody show is thick, mucousy, and pink or dark red. Active vaginal bleeding is thin, watery, and bright red.

6. *Placenta previa* is a condition in which the placenta abnormally implants in the lower uterine wall.

7. *Abruptio placentae* is a condition in which a normally implanted placenta prematurely separates from the uterine wall.

8. *Amniotomy* is a procedure by which the membranes are artificially ruptured.

9. The significance of meconium-stained amniotic fluid is:
   a. Meconium-stained amniotic fluid when the fetus presents head first indicates fetal anoxia (distress).
   b. Meconium-stained amniotic fluid when the fetus presents buttocks first is normal.

10. *Hydramnios or polyhydramnios* is an excessive amount of amniotic fluid associated with malformations in which the fetus is usually unable to swallow and urinate normally in utero.

11. Three tests commonly used to document ROM are:
    a. *Nitrazine test tape.* Amniotic fluid changes the pH causing the tape to change to blue-green, blue-grey, or dark blue.
    b. *Staining of fetal fat cells.* Nile blue sulfate added to amniotic fluid causes fetal fat cells to stain orange.
    c. *Ferning of cervical mucus.* Cervical mucus mixed with amniotic fluid changes to a fernlike pattern of crystallization.

Stages of Labor

STAGE I. The stage of dilatation begins with the onset of regular contractions and ends with complete cervical dilatation and effacement. Stage I is divided into three phases. (See Chapter 4.) The average length of time is 12½ to 14 hours for the primigravida and 6 to 7½ hours for the multigravida.

STAGE II. The stage of expulsion begins with complete dilatation and ends with delivery of the baby. The average length of time is 1½ hours for the primigravida and ½ hour for the multigravida. Although the woman has been in labor for many hours up to this point, Stage II is the actual working stage. She must actively push with contractions to assist the movement of the baby through the birth canal.

STAGE III. The placental stage begins with delivery of the baby and ends with expulsion of the placenta. The average length of time is 20 minutes (⅓ hour).

STAGE IV. The recovery stage is the first 1 to 4 hours after delivery of the placenta.

Review Question

Using the chart on page 11, indicate the beginning and end of each stage of labor. Include the approximate duration of labor for the primigravida (P) and the multigravida (M).

Stage	Begins With	Ends With	Hours Duration	
			P	M
I				
II				
III				
IV				

Answer

Stage	Begins With	Ends With	Hours Duration	
			P	M
I	regular contractions	complete dilatation and effacement	12½–14	6–7½
II	complete dilatation	delivery of the baby	1½	½
III	delivery of the baby	delivery of the placenta	⅓	⅓
IV	delivery of the placenta	1–4 hours after delivery of the placenta	1–4	1–4

Fetal Relationship to Maternal Pelvis

FETAL LIE. Lie refers to the relationship of the longitudinal axis (head to feet) of the fetus to the longitudinal axis of the mother. Ninety-nine percent of all lies are longitudinal; that is, the baby's longitudinal axis is parallel with the mother's. One percent are perpendicular, known as a transverse lie (shoulder presentation).

FETAL ATTITUDE. Attitude refers to the relationship of the fetal parts to each other—the degree of flexion or extension. The normal fetal attitude is one of moderate flexion. The chin is flexed on the chest, and the extremities are flexed on the abdomen, thereby taking up the smallest possible space in utero.

PRESENTATION. Presentation refers to that part of the fetus that is lowermost in the pelvis. The part that first enters the pelvis is the presenting part. The most common presentation (95 percent) is cephalic (head). The degree of flexion or extension determines the type of cephalic presentation (Fig. 1-1). Cephalic presentations include the following variations.

Occipital or vertex presentation occurs when the head is fully flexed on the chest so that the occiput (O) is the presenting part in the lower segment of the uterus. This is the ideal presentation. *Sinciput* presentation (military attitude) occurs when the head is neither flexed nor extended so that the anterior fontanel is the presenting part. This usually reverts to an occipital presentation for delivery. *Brow* presentation occurs when the head is extended so that the forehead (brow—B) is the presenting part. A *face* or *chin* presentation occurs when the head is hyperextended so that the chin (mentum—M) is the presenting part.

Presentations in which the lower body parts present first are termed *breech* and occur in 3 percent of term deliveries. There are three types of breech presentations. In a *frank breech,* the presenting part is the buttocks with the thighs flexed on the abdomen and the legs extended onto the chest. A *complete breech* is characterized by flexion of the thighs on the abdomen and flexion of the calves on the thighs. In a single (or double) *footling breech,* one leg (or both) is extended at the knees and hips.

A *shoulder* presentation occurs when the fetus is in a transverse lie. The scapula (Sc) is the presenting part. Vaginal delivery is not possible unless the fetus can be rotated to a longitudinal lie. If rotation is not possible, cesarean delivery is necessary. This presentation is rare.

POSITION. Position is the relationship between the presenting part of the fetus and the maternal pelvis. The maternal pelvis is divided into four

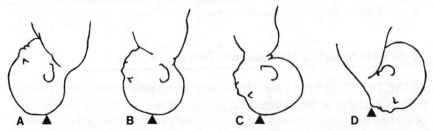

Figure 1-1. Cephalic (head) presentations. (*A*) Occipital or vertex; (*B*) sinciput; (*C*) brow; and (*D*) face or chin.

TABLE 1-1   Fetal Lie, Presentation, Presenting Part, and Position

LIE Presentation	Presenting Part	Sample Position
LONGITUDINAL		
Cephalic		
a. Vertex	Occiput (O)*	Left Occiput Anterior (LOA)
b. Brow	Brow (B)*	Right Brow Posterior (RBP)
c. Face	Mentum (M)*	Left Mentum Anterior (LMA)
Breech	Sacrum (S)*	Right Sacrum Posterior (RSP)
TRANSVERSE		
Shoulder	Scapula (Sc)*	Left Scapula Anterior (LScA)

*Symbol for presenting part used in position

quadrants: left anterior, left posterior, right anterior, and right posterior. In a vertex presentation, if the occiput is directed toward the left anterior quadrant of the pelvis, then the fetal position is left occiput anterior (LOA). See Table 1-1 for examples of fetal positions as they relate to lie, presentation, and presenting part.

STATION. The assessment of the level of descent of the presenting part in relation to the ischial spines of the maternal pelvis is termed *station*. When the presenting part, the bony prominence of the head, is at the level of the ischial spines, the station is zero (0), and engagement has occurred. The presenting part is said to be floating when it is entirely out of the pelvis and freely movable. The progression of descent is measured in centimeters moving from a negative to a positive station designated as -5 (at the level of the pelvic inlet), $-4, \ldots 0 \ldots +4, +5$ (pelvic outlet).

Review Questions

1. The relationship of the longitudinal axis of the fetus to the longitudinal axis of the mother is termed _____ .

2. The relationship of the fetal parts to each other is called _____ _____ .

3. Define presentation. _____
_____
_____

4. The most common presentation is _____ .

5. Briefly describe the three types of breech presentations.

   a. _____
   _____
   _____

   b. _____
   _____
   _____

   c. _____
   _____
   _____

6. Write in the correct name of the presenting part for each of the following presentations:

Presentation	Presenting Part
Cephalic: Vertex	
Brow	
Face	
Breech	
Shoulder	

7. The relationship of the presenting part of the fetus to the maternal pelvis is called _____ .

8. Fetal descent is assessed in relation to the ischial spines of the maternal pelvis. This is called _____ .

9. Define the term floating. _____
   _____
   _____

Answers

1. *Lie* is the relationship of the longitudinal axis of the fetus to the longitudinal axis of the mother.

2. *Attitude* is the relationship of the fetal parts to each other.

3. Presentation refers to the part of the fetus that is lowermost in the pelvis.

4. The most common presentation is *cephalic (head); occipital (vertex).*

5. Three types of breech presentations are:
    a. Frank breech—thighs flexed on the abdomen with legs extended onto the chest.
    b. Complete breech—thighs flexed on the abdomen and calves flexed on the thighs.
    c. Footling breech—one or both legs extended at the knees and hips.

6. The presenting part for each of the following presentations is:

Presentation	Presenting Part
Cephalic: Vertex	Occiput
Brow	Brow
Face	Mentum
Breech	Sacrum
Shoulder	Scapula

7. *Position* is the relationship of the presenting part of the fetus to the maternal pelvis.

8. *Station* is the assessment of fetal descent in relation to the ischial spines of the maternal pelvis.

9. The presenting part is floating when it is freely movable above the pelvic inlet; above −5 station; not engaged.

Mechanisms of Labor

The mechanisms of labor are sequential maneuvers within the maternal pelvis that the fetus must accomplish so that vaginal delivery can occur. (See Chapter 3 for a more in-depth description.)

DESCENT. Initial descent occurs simultaneously with engagement. The head enters the pelvis with the occiput transverse (to the side) in the pelvic inlet. The fetus descends during each contraction and slightly retracts during relaxation so that the progression is slow.

FLEXION. As the fetal head encounters resistance from the maternal pelvis it flexes so that a smaller diameter of the head presents.

INTERNAL ROTATION. The fetal head rotates from occiput transverse to occiput anterior (45 degrees), which places the occiput beneath the symphysis pubis.

EXTENSION. The head is born during extension. First emerges the occiput, then the face, then the chin.

RESTITUTION, EXTERNAL ROTATION, AND EXPULSION. Once the head is delivered and free from pressure and compression, it immediately rotates *(restitution)* 45 degrees back to the transverse position. The head then rotates *(external rotation)* another 45 degrees, placing the shoulders in the anterior-posterior diameter. The rest of the baby, which is smaller in diameter, is delivered spontaneously *(expulsion)*.

Review Questions

Circle True or False and explain your answer.

1. T   F   The correct sequence of the mechanisms of labor is descent, flexion, extension, internal rotation, restitution, external rotation, expulsion.

2. T   F   Descent occurs simultaneously with engagement.

3. T   F   Restitution occurs as the head encounters resistance from the maternal pelvis.

Answers

1. *False.*   Internal rotation must occur before the baby's head can be born during extension.

2. *True.*   Initial descent occurs simultaneously with engagement.

3. *False.*   Flexion occurs as the head encounters resistance from the maternal pelvis. Restitution is the process of rotating 45 degrees back to the transverse position after delivery of the head.

NURSING CARE DURING THE LABOR AND DELIVERY PROCESS

Recognition of the Onset of Labor

During the latter part of pregnancy, the woman should be taught to recognize the premonitory signs of labor. In review, they are engagement, uterine contractions, cervical changes, bloody show, rupture of membranes, sudden burst of energy, increased backache, increased vaginal secretions, sudden 2 to 3 pound weight loss, and loose stools or diarrhea. She should notify her physician when uterine contractions felt primarily in the lower back are regular, are 5 to 10 minutes apart and last at least 30 seconds, and continue despite walking. If membranes rupture spontaneously with or without contractions, the woman is usually advised to report to the hospital as soon as possible. Nursing care of the labor patient begins with the first verbal contact, usually a telephone notification that the patient is coming to the hospital.

It is important for the nurse to review the patient's prenatal record for significant data prior to admission. She should assess the following areas:
1. Obstetric History
   a. Estimated date of confinement (EDC); Age; Gravida; Para; Abortions; Stillbirths; Neonatal deaths; Living children (G_____ , P_____ , Ab_____ , SB_____ , ND_____ , LC_____ ,)
   b. Pregnancy course: maternal vital signs, fetal heart rate, fundal growth pattern, complications such as toxemia, gestational diabetes, infections (TORCH*), abnormal weight gain
   c. Lab results: urine (protein, ketones, glucose) and blood (hemaglobin/hematocrit, Type and Rh, VDRL, titers)
   d. Previous obstetric complications related to pregnancy, labor, or delivery
2. Medical history: conditions that would place the mother and/or fetus/ newborn at risk. (See Chapter 9.)
3. Other Pertinent Information
   a. Method of preparation for labor/delivery
   b. Analgesia/anesthesia preference
   c. Birth preferences
   d. Cultural, religious, or ethnic influences
   e. Marital status

---

*Toxoplasmosis, Other, Rubella, Cytomegalovirus, Herpes.

f. Anxieties or fears

g. Plans for breast or bottle feeding.

If the woman has not received prenatal care, or if her records are unavailable, the above information will need to be obtained at the time of admission.

Initial Assessment

The initial assessment by the nurse or physician is performed to determine if the woman is in labor, how far she has progressed, and her initial psychologic response to labor. She may prefer to have her support person remain in the room during the assessment. Assistance may be needed to undress and put on a hospital gown. This is a good time to obtain a urine specimen for urinalysis, protein, ketones, and glucose. An empty bladder further facilitates examination and causes the woman less discomfort. Vital signs are obtained for comparison with the prenatal baseline. Occasionally, the excitement of coming to the hospital may cause the systolic blood pressure (BP) to be slightly elevated. If this occurs, the procedure should be repeated in 15 to 30 minutes for a more accurate reading.

Evaluation begins with assessment of the contractions. Ask the woman to describe her contractions. Where does she feel them? How do they feel? When did they begin? How frequently do they occur and how long do they last? Palpate her contractions and compare what you feel with her perceptions. (See Chapter 2).

LEOPOLD'S MANEUVERS. Fetal position and presentation can be determined manually using Leopold's Maneuvers (Fig. 1-2). With the woman in a supine position, drapes are applied so that the abdomen is exposed. The following four maneuvers are performed.

First Maneuver. Place both hands on the fundus and palpate to determine the contents. The head is firm, round, and freely movable. In a cephalic presentation, the buttocks should be identifiable in the fundus.

Second Maneuver. Move both hands concurrently down both sides of the abdomen to determine on which side of the uterus the fetal back lies. One hand remains stationary while the other palpates. The fetal back is identified as a smooth, curved, resistant plane. Opposite the back are the fetal front surface (concave and soft) and small parts, that is, feet, hands, elbows, knees (irregular projections).

Third Maneuver. Gently grasp the bottom of the uterus, pressing in slightly with thumb and fingers to determine which fetal part is present-

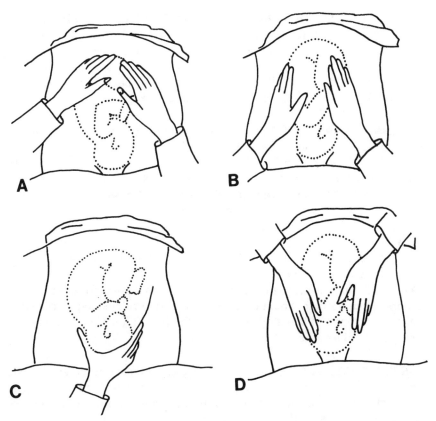

Figure 1-2. Leopold's maneuvers. (*A*) First; (*B*) second; (*C*) third; and (*D*) fourth.

ing over the pelvic inlet. If the head is the presenting part, it will feel round and hard. If engagement has not occurred, the head can be gently rocked from side to side. The presence of the fetal head at the pelvic inlet provides the following information: longitudinal lie and cephalic presentation.

Fourth Maneuver. Stand near the woman's shoulders and face her feet. With the fingers of both hands, press in two inches on both sides of the abdomen just above the symphysis pubis. Exert gentle pressure downward (towards her feet). If one hand meets firm resistance, this is probably the fetal brow. If the fetal brow is felt on the same side as the small parts, then the head is well flexed. Only a small portion of the presenting part may be palpable if it has descended deeply into the pelvic inlet, that is, if engagement has occurred.

AUSCULTATION OF FETAL HEART RATE (FHR). The FHR is best heard through the fetal back in a vertex or breech presentation, and through the chest in a face presentation. In a vertex presentation, one would listen to the FHR below the maternal umbilicus on either the left or the right side, depending on where the fetal back is located. (See Chapter 2 for further discussion of assessing FHR.)

VAGINAL EXAMINATIONS. Vaginal examinations are performed gently, using aseptic technique. Palpation of the cervix provides dilatation and effacement data. Through a dilating cervix, the examiner will be able to determine fetal presentation (cephalic, breech, shoulder), station (degree of descent in relation to the ischial spines), and position. If the bag of waters is felt, this indicates that the membranes are intact. General assessment of the pelvis may also be performed at this time. (See Chapter 3). The frequency of vaginal exams will be determined by labor progress. Vaginal exams should be kept to a minimum. Instruct the patient about the procedure to decrease anxiety and promote relaxation. It is important to share findings with the laboring couple so that they are aware of the progress being made. Vaginal exams may be contraindicated in the presence of any vaginal bleeding because of the possibility of placenta previa or abruptio placentae.

X-RAY/ULTRASOUND. X-ray pelvimetry can be used to determine the presentation, position, lie, and attitude of the fetus. This may be necessary only when manual examination is inconclusive. Since the effects of radiographic rays on the maternal ovaries and the fetus are not known, caution should be used in making the decision. According to Oxorn and Foote,[2] valid indications for pelvimetry include (1) previous difficult delivery; (2) abnormal or grossly contracted pelvis; (3) breech presentation; or (4) abnormal progress in second stage, undiagnosed fetal position, attitude, and station. A definite diagnosis of the above with pelvimetry would provide early indications for changing the management of labor and delivery.

Fetal presentation and position can also be determined from *pulsed-echo ultrasound*. This procedure has replaced the use of X-ray pelvimetry in many institutions. High frequency sound waves are used to scan the mother's abdomen. The procedure is noninvasive and painless. There are no known contraindications to the use of ultrasound. (See Chapter 6.)

Following the initial assessment, if the woman is thought to be in labor, she should be admitted to the labor unit. If she is not in true labor, she may be sent home. If the distance is great, she may be asked to walk around for an hour and return for re-examination. If the woman is sent home, this can create feelings of great disappointment, which the nurse needs to understand.

Review Questions

1. Mrs. Brown calls the labor unit and states that her membranes ruptured but she is not in labor. The best response by the nurse would be:
   a. "You need to wait until your contractions start before coming to the hospital."
   b. "Come to the hospital as soon as possible so the doctor can check you and your baby."
   c. "Why don't you wait a few hours and call me back if anything happens."
   d. "You can come to the hospital if you want to, but it will be awhile before your baby is born."

2. According to Mrs. Black's prenatal chart she is G-vii, P-iv, Ab-ii, SB-i. Therefore, you might assume that Mrs. Black has experienced labor and delivery _____ number of times.

3. During the initial assessment, urine is usually tested for which of the following?
   a. Protein, Hemaglobin, Rh
   b. VDRL, Ketones, Hemaglobin
   c. Rh, VDRL, Glucose
   d. Protein, Ketones, Glucose

4. Using Leopold's maneuvers, in a cephalic presentation the buttocks should be identifiable in the _____ .

5. The FHR is best heard through the fetal back in a _____ _____ or _____ presentation.

6. Vaginal exams may be contraindicated in the presence of _____ _____ .

7. List three situations in which the use of X-ray pelvimetry is considered valid even though the effects of radiographic rays are unknown.
   a. _____
   b. _____
   c. _____

Answers

1. <u>b</u>. If membranes rupture spontaneously, with or without contractions, the woman is usually advised to report to the hospital as soon as possible for assessment of fetal well-being.

2. Mrs. Black has experienced labor and delivery 4 times. This is Mrs. Black's 7th pregnancy (G-vii). She has had 6 previous pregnancies.

Two of them were aborted (*Ab-ii*) and *one* resulted in a stillbirth (*SB-i*).

3. $\underline{d}$. Urine is tested for protein, ketones, and glucose.

4. Using Leopold's maneuvers, in a cephalic presentation the buttocks should be identifiable in the *fundus*.

5. The FHR is best heard through the fetal back in a *vertex* or *breech* presentation.

6. Vaginal exams may be contraindicated in the presence of *vaginal bleeding*.

7. Situations in which the use of pelvimetry is considered valid include (a) previous difficult delivery; (b) abnormal or grossly contracted pelvis; (c) breech presentation; or (d) abnormal progress in second stage, undiagnosed fetal position, attitude, and station.

Latent Phase of the First Stage of Labor

During the latent phase of the first stage of labor progress is slow. The cervix dilates from 1 to 3 cm. Effacement is often complete before dilatation begins in the primigravida and occurs simultaneously with dilatation in the multigravida. Contractions are usually mild and may be irregular with a frequency of 5 to 20 minutes. The duration is 10 to 30 seconds.

The woman may be excited and talkative. She cannot believe labor has finally begun. She might be quiet and afraid. Although she wants the baby, she may not feel ready for labor and would like to make it go away. She and her husband (or significant other) may have some fear of the unknown and are usually open to instruction and directions.

EMOTIONAL FEARS COMMONLY ASSOCIATED WITH CHILDBIRTH. Women who experience unresolved fear during labor are more likely to have increased tension and prolonged labor. Fears commonly associated with childbirth fall into two categories: fears the woman has about herself and fears about the baby.

Fears the woman might have about herself include:
1. A fear of pain: pain associated with labor, delivery, examinations, needles.
2. A fear of long labor: if the labor is too long, she won't be able to stand the pain; she might hemorrhage.
3. A fear of abandonment during labor: she might be left alone, and because she won't know what to do terrible things might happen to her and/or the baby.

4. A fear of being internally injured or torn: perhaps she thinks she is too small; intrusive procedures could cause injury.
5. A fear of losing self-esteem: doubtfulness of her ability to cope during labor; fear of losing control, making a fool of herself, and thereby alienating her partner.
6. A fear of embarrassment: nudity; urinating and defecating in bed; messiness from amniotic fluid and vaginal discharge; foul language.
7. Fears of helplessness; unable to control the onset or progress of labor; unable to control what others do to her during labor and delivery.

Fears the woman might have about the baby include:
1. Fear that the baby might not survive the labor/delivery process.
2. Fear that the baby might be injured during the delivery.
3. Fear that the baby will have gross deformities.
4. Fear that the baby won't come out at all and if it does, fears about how it will get out.

These fears may be reduced by:[3]
1. Explaining the process of labor to the unprepared mother in terms she understands and reviewing the process with educationally prepared couples. Review emotions and sensations the mother is likely to experience as labor progresses.
2. Keeping parents informed as labor progresses. Provide parents with opportunities for validation of health and progress, e.g, listening to the fetal heart beat.
3. Praising and reinforcing the mother's efforts to cope, and using this method of teaching to modify inappropriate behavior. Animate desired breathing patterns with the patient, if necessary, i.e., perform breathing exercises with her during contractions.
4. Providing physically supportive care, thereby decreasing her discomfort and building upon rapport and trust in the nurse. Some physical comfort measures include: comfortable positioning, back rubs, effleurage (a form of light, lower abdominal massage), appropriate coaching during and between contractions, wiping perspiration with a cool damp cloth, periodic mouth rinses, and the application of lip emollients.

ORIENTATION TO ENVIRONMENT. Admission usually occurs during early labor. Orientation to the unit and the labor room will make the couple feel more welcome. Allow the woman to familiarize herself with her surroundings by walking around the room, sitting in a chair, and so forth. If she is tired and needs to rest, then encourage a side-lying position to facilitate placental oxygenation. This is a good time to get to know the couple and explore their preparation and anticipations about their labor and delivery. Explain the purpose of the call light and place it within easy reach when you leave the room.

PERINEAL PREPARATION. A wide range of preps may be used from a full perineal shave to just clipping the hair. If shaving is practiced, avoid creating skin nicks with the razor. These become sites for infection. Some institutions allow just a thorough cleansing of the perianal area. Throughout labor, the perineum should be kept as clean and dry as possible.

VITAL SIGNS. Maternal vital signs provide data on the state of hydration and maternal/fetal status. The temperature should be taken every 4 hours throughout labor, unless it is greater than 37.2°C (99.0°F), in which case it should be taken at least every 2 hours. This routine may be altered following ROM. (See Chapter 5.) Check blood pressure and pulse every 1 to 2 hours, unless the BP is greater than 140/90 or the pulse is greater than 100 beats per minute. In these cases more frequent assessment is necessary.

FETAL HEART RATE. FHR provides information for evaluating fetal response to labor and fetal well-being. FHR should be assessed at least every 30 minutes throughout the first stage of labor as long as it remains between 120 to 160 beats per minute. (See Chapter 2.)

CONTRACTIONS. Palpate contractions and compare your assessment (see Chapter 2) with the woman's perception of what she is feeling. Observe her reactions. If she is expending too much energy, this is a good time to evaluate and possibly change her coping behaviors.

ACTIVITY. Hospital policies will vary, but generally the woman may walk around or be in bed as she desires, provided all of the following are present: (1) uncomplicated pregnancy; (2) good fetal response to labor; (3) normal presentation; and (4) engagement. Provide diversional activities and encourage the woman to relax. The couple usually functions well independently during this early (latent) phase; however, the nurse should create opportunities for answering questions and giving information.

NUTRITION. Solid foods are not recommended during labor because of decreased gastrointestinal absorption. However, clear liquids and ice chips provide energy and maintain hydration. If the woman becomes dehydrated and is experiencing nausea or vomiting during labor, fluids may need to be given intravenously. If a cesarean delivery is anticipated, oral fluids should not be given.

ELIMINATION. A full bladder can interfere with the progress of labor and with descent of the fetus and cause discomfort. Assess the bladder status every 2 hours during labor. Hormones of pregnancy, pressure from the presenting part, and analgesia may cause decreased bladder tone so that the urge to void is not present. Encourage the woman to void as necessary. When she does, the amount should be recorded and the urine should be tested for protein, ketones, and glucose.

It is no longer routine to give every patient in labor an *enema*. However, if the woman has not had a bowel movement during the last 24 hours or if fecal matter is felt in the rectum during examination, an enema may be indicated. Removing stool from the lower bowel facilitates descent of the presenting part. (See Chapter 5.)

COMFORT MEASURES. Continual assessment throughout labor will determine the type and amount of comfort measures needed. Prepared and experienced couples may only need reinforcement of what they were taught prior to labor. Inexperienced couples may need additional suggestions.

Position is probably the most important aspect of comfort. Whether the woman is standing, sitting, or lying down, she will need support to maintain her position during contractions. Pillows can be used to support the upper and lower back, head, and arms. (See Chapters 3 and 9). Frequent position changes should be encouraged throughout labor; however, the woman should avoid the supine position, which may interfere with oxygenation of the placenta and consequently the fetus.

Conscious relaxation, breathing techniques, effleurage, pelvic rock, heat to the lower back, back rubs, and counterpressure on the lower back all provide an alternative focus to decrease perception of pain with contractions. (See Chapter 8.) Couples should be taught to expend as little energy as possible in promoting comfort during labor.

Dry mouth and cracked lips can be very uncomfortable. Frequent fluids or ice chips help. Lemon and glycerine swabs or lollipops provide additional lubrication. Frequent mouth rinses help remove the bad taste that accompanies a dry mouth.

Comfort measures may not always be effective in decreasing the perception of pain. Medicinal intervention may become necessary to facilitate coping and promote labor progression. (See Chapter 7.)

Review Questions

1. Complete the chart on page 26 with the appropriate descriptive words for the latent phase of the first stage of labor.

	Latent Phase
Dilatation	
Contraction: frequency	
duration	
intensity	

2. Identify three fears a woman in labor might have about herself and three fears she might have about her baby.
    a. Fears the woman might have about herself:
        1. _____
        2. _____
        3. _____
    b. Fears the woman might have about the baby:
        1. _____
        2. _____
        3. _____

Answers

1.

	Latent Phase
Dilatation	1–3 cm
Contraction: frequency	5–20 minutes
duration	10–30 seconds
intensity	mild

2. a. Fears the woman might have about herself:
    1. pain
    2. long labor
    3. abandonment
    4. internal injury
    5. losing self-esteem
    6. embarrassment
    7. helplessness

    b. Fears the woman might have about the baby: 1. survival; 2. injury; 3. deformities; 4. the baby won't come out or fear about how the baby will get out.

Early Active Phase of the First Stage of Labor

During the active (acceleration) phase of the first stage of labor, progress becomes more rapid. The cervix dilates from 4 to 7 cm. Effacement is probably complete. Contractions are usually regular, are moderate in intensity, occur every 3 to 5 minutes, and last 30 to 45 seconds. Increased bloody show and vaginal discharge are present.

The woman may become apprehensive. She becomes doubtful of her ability to control the pain. She may be afraid to be alone. Her attention becomes more inner-directed. She may have difficulty following directions. Fatigue is evident.

Upon entering the room the nurse should not interrupt the couple's concentration during contractions. Evaluate the effectiveness of their coping mechanisms. Praise the couple's positive efforts. Offer to relieve the coach from time to time to decrease his fatigue. Provide an environment that is conducive to rest and relaxation. Encourage complete relaxation between contractions. This will conserve energy and promote labor. Physical nursing care (vital signs, FHR, contractions, nutrition, elimination, comfort measures) must be provided but with minimal disruption for the couple.

Transition Phase of the First Stage of Labor

During the transition (maximum slope) phase of labor, progress is most rapid. The cervix dilates from 8 to 10 cm. Contractions are usually regular and strong to expulsive and occur every 2 to 3 minutes and last 45 to 60 seconds. Bloody show is heavy and intact membranes may rupture spontaneously.

The woman will often lose control during transition. Irritability may take the form of anger or unwillingness to be touched. Communication is brief with periods of amnesia between contractions. Response to contractions may include writhing, nausea and vomiting, and hyperventilation. Profuse perspiration (diaphoresis) occurs. She may also experience muscle cramps, leg tremors, and generalized shaking. The urge to defecate is strong because of pressure on the anus. This is experienced as an urge to push or bear down. Pain is described as severe, and many women express the feeling of not being able to make it. If ever they need support it is now.

The primigravida will stay in the labor room through transition and until the fetus has descended so that the perineal area is bulging. The multigravida may be taken to the delivery room at the beginning of transition (8 cm), since tissue and muscles of the birth canal are more relaxed from previous births. Accomplish the transfer with as little disruption as possible.

Regardless of where she is, continue to assess maternal vital signs and FHR. Evaluate each contraction using very light touch without pressure. Encourage and assist with position changes, keeping the perianal area as clean and dry as possible. If severe back pain is present, firm pressure and/or heat may be applied. Nausea and vomiting may be alleviated with a cold wet cloth placed on the neck. Frequent facial wipes and mouth care promote comfort. (See Chapters 8 and 9 for other supportive techniques.) Regardless of how strong the urge, pushing should not be allowed until the cervix is completely dilated. Panting through each contraction helps to overcome the urge to push.

Review Questions

1. Complete the following chart with the appropriate descriptive words for the early active phase and transition phase of the first stage of labor.

	Early Active Phase	Transition
Dilatation		
Contraction: frequency		
duration		
intensity		

2. Match the terms in column I with the appropriate phase of labor, in column II.

Column I	Column II
a. Latent phase	__ Irritable, unwilling to be touched.
b. Early active phase	__ Strong urge to push or bear down.
	__ Becomes doubtful of ability to control pain.
c. Transition phase	__ May not feel ready for labor.
	__ May be afraid to be alone.
	__ Open to instructions and directions.
	__ Periods of amnesia occur between contractions.
	__ Fatigue becomes evident.
	__ Period when the woman needs the most support.

Answers

1.

	Early Active Phase	Transition
Dilatation	4–7 cm	8–10 cm
Contraction: frequency	3–5 min	2–3 min
duration	30–45 sec	45–60 sec
intensity	moderate	strong–expulsive

2. c, c, b, a, b, a, c, b, c.

During the *latent phase* the following may occur: may not feel ready for labor; open to instructions and directions.

During the *early active phase* the following may occur: becomes doubtful of ability to control pain; may be afraid to be alone; fatigue becomes evident.

During the *transition phase* the following may occur: irritable, unwilling to be touched; strong urge to push or bear down; periods of amnesia occur between contractions; period when the woman needs the most support.

Second Stage of Labor

Labor is the expenditure of energy to accomplish delivery. The period of greatest energy flow is the second stage, the stage of expulsion. During the second stage, uterine contractions usually occur every 2 to 3 minutes, last 50 to 60 seconds, and are expulsive in strength. The urge to push or bear down is very strong. Coordinating involuntary uterine contractions and the voluntary contractions of pushing will promote progressive descent with crowning and delivery of the baby.

The couple is usually excited about the prospect of imminent delivery. If fatigue or discouragement have been present, they will usually disappear with a new surge of hope and feelings of positive accomplishment.

The nurse should monitor each contraction. FHR should be taken after each contraction or every 5 minutes. Continuous pressure is exerted on the fetal head during descent through the vaginal canal. A drop in FHR may require turning the woman on her side or facilitating immediate delivery. Blood pressure and pulse are taken every 15 minutes and should be done between contractions.

Cervical dilatation, effacement, and descent of the presenting part are determined by vaginal examination. The cervix must be completely dilated before pushing is allowed or encouraged. Pushing prior to complete dilatation may cause edema of the portion of the cervix that is not dilated and thereby prolong labor. (See Chapter 9 for discussion of coaching and positions for pushing.) Pushing is encouraged until the presenting part (fetal head) is visible at the vaginal opening (introitus) with each contraction. If an episiotomy (surgical incision) is necessary to enlarge the vaginal opening, it will be performed at this time. (See Chapter 7 for anesthetics used at the time of delivery.) The woman may be encouraged to pant (stop pushing) so that the head is delivered gently with only the power of involuntary uterine contractions.

If a delivery room birth is planned, transfer should be as nonintrusive as possible. Most hospitals are now equipped with labor beds that can be used for transport, thus omitting the necessity of having the woman move to a stretcher. The practice of rushing to the delivery room while repeatedly telling the woman "don't push" causes a great deal of anxiety. This can be omitted through careful planning and monitoring of labor progression. Delivery may be accomplished on either the labor bed or the delivery table. If the delivery table is used, transfer from the bed should be done in between contractions.

In the delivery room the nurse should show the father where to sit or stand in order to continue coaching and observe the birth if he chooses. In addition to continual assessment of maternal/fetal status, the nurse must also prepare the mother physically. Support her head and shoulders with pillows, place her legs in stirrups, and cleanse the perianal area. Instruct the woman to grasp the handles on the table. Strapping her hands to the table is not usually necessary. Instruct her not to touch the sterile field. The nurse also needs to prepare the equipment for the delivery and assist the physician to don sterile gown and gloves.

Third Stage of Labor

The newborn is usually placed on the mother's abdomen immediately after delivery for clamping and cutting the cord. However, the newborn should be placed at the level of the uterus prior to clamping the cord. This prevents blood loss to the placenta when the baby is held above the uterus or an increased amount of blood from the placenta to the newborn when the baby is held below the level of the uterus. Whether to clamp the cord immediately or wait for pulsations to cease is controversial.

Parents' reactions to this first sight of their baby are varied. They may stare in awe, scream, shout, laugh, or cry. The excitement is usually high. They involuntarily reach out to touch the baby. Occasionaly, disappointment over the sex of the baby may be verbally expressed. The nurse should be accepting of all feelings that occur at this time. (Nursing care of the newborn immediately after delivery will be discussed later.)

The third stage, the placental stage, is very short. It involves passively waiting for placental separation. The signs of placental separation are: (1) the uterus becomes more global in shape and rises in the abdominal cavity; (2) the cord visibly lengthens outside the vagina; and (3) a trickle or gush of bright red blood exits the vaginal canal. Following signs of separation, the woman may be asked to push or bear down to facilitate placental expulsion.

The nurse may receive an order to administer an oxytocic drug (Pitocin, Methergine, Syntocinon) immediately following delivery of the placenta. Oxytocics stimulate uterine contractions and decrease blood loss from the placental implantation site. An oxytocic may be administered earlier with the delivery of the anterior shoulder of the newborn for the same purpose.

Delivery of the placenta followed by the contraction or clamping down of the uterus may be painful and unexpected by the mother. Support and reassurance are important during this time.

Fourth Stage of Labor

Following examination of the vagina and cervix, and episiotomy repair if necessary, the mother is transferred to the recovery area. Positive identification of mother and baby must be done before the transfer.

Nursing assessment of the mother is done every 15 minutes during the first hour and every 30 minutes for at least 1 to 2 hours. Nursing assessment includes:

Vital Signs. Blood pressure and pulse provide significant data regarding the new mother's circulatory status. They are initially assessed every 15 minutes. The temperature should be taken at least once during the recovery period, unless predisposing factors for infection have occurred. In that case the temperature should be taken every 2 hours.

Fundus. The fundus should be firm, midline, and at the level of or below the umbilicus. If it is not firm, massage is indicated to prevent hemorrhage at the placental implantation site. If clots are present, they must be expressed if the fundus is to remain firm. If the fundus is not firm, or if it is above the umbilicus and/or deviated from midline, bladder distention should be suspected.

Lochia. Check for color, amount, and presence of clots. Lochia should be red and moderate in amount. Saturating one pad during the period of an hour constitutes normal lochia flow during Stage IV. The presence of solid particles may indicate retained placental fragments or relaxation of the fundus. A cervical laceration may be suspected if the lochia flows in spurts or continuously trickles in the presence of a firm fundus.

Perineum. Whether or not an episiotomy has been performed, the perineum should be inspected for signs of excess trauma, swelling, bruising, or tears. Some edema may occur following episiotomy repair. Intermittent ice to the perineum during the first 24 hours postpartum will help prevent undue bruising, swelling, and pain.

Urinary Bladder. Immediately following delivery, the bladder has increased capacity, decreased tone, and decreased sensitivity. The bladder should be palpated for urinary retention and the patient encouraged to void as necessary. Catheterization may be necessary.

Review Questions

1. The period of greatest energy flow for the woman in labor is the _____ stage of labor.

2. Pushing is allowed/encouraged when the cervix is dilated:
   a. 5 cm   b. 7 cm   c. 9 cm   d. 10 cm

3. A surgical incision sometimes used to enlarge the vaginal opening is an _____ .

4. List three components of nursing assessment of maternal/fetal status during the second stage of labor:
   a. _____
   b. _____
   c. _____

5. List three signs of placental separation:
   a. _____
   b. _____
   c. _____

6. All *but one* of the following drugs are oxytocics used to stimulate uterine contractions and may be administered following delivery of the placenta:
   a. Pitocin   b. Methergine   c. Aquamephyton   d. Syntocinon

7. Following delivery, the fundus is assessed *every* 15 minutes during the first hour. It should be firm and:
   a.   midline and above the umbilicus
   b.   midline and at the level of the umbilicus
   c.   deviated to the right and above the umbilicus
   d.   deviated to the right and at the level of the umbilicus

8. Following episiotomy repair, perineal bruising, swelling, and pain can be decreased with the application of _____ .

9. Which of the following has increased capacity, decreased tone, and decreased sensitivity following delivery?
   a. pituitary gland   b. liver   c. urinary bladder   d. heart

Answers

1. The *second* stage of labor is the period of greatest energy flow for the woman in labor.

2. d. Pushing is allowed/encouraged when the cervix is dilated 10 cm.

3. *Episiotomy* is a surgical incision sometimes used to enlarge the vaginal opening.

4. Nursing assessment of maternal/fetal status during the second stage of labor includes: (a) continuous monitoring of contractions; (b) FHR after every contraction or every 5 minutes; and (c) blood pressure and pulse every 15 minutes.

5. Three signs of placental separation are: (a) the uterus becomes more global in shape and rises in the abdomen; (b) the cord visibly lengthens outside the vagina; and (c) a trickle or gush of bright red blood exits the vagina.

6. c. Aquamephyton is not an oxytocic drug. Pitocin, Methergine, and Syntocinon are all oxytocics.

7. b. Following delivery the fundus should be firm, midline, and at or below the level of the umbilicus.

8. *Ice* applied to the perineum after episiotomy repair will decrease bruising, swelling, and pain.

9. c. The urinary bladder has increased capacity, decreased tone, and decreased sensitivity following delivery.

Immediate Nursing Care of the Newborn

As soon as delivery is complete, a timer should be set for one minute and five minutes to obtain Apgar scores. The Apgar score chart (Table 1-2) was developed by Dr. Virginia Apgar as a method of evaluating the newborn's adaptation from intrauterine to extrauterine environment at one minute after birth. The five-minute score evaluates the newborn's responsiveness to resuscitation measures. A score of 7 to 10 means good condition; 3 to 6 means moderately depressed; and 0 to 2 means severely depressed. Resuscitative measures are indicated if the score is less than 7. There is a direct correlation between the five-minute Apgar score and newborn morbidity/mortality.

The newborn should be dried immediately and placed under a radiant warmer or skin to skin with mother and covered with warm blankets to prevent heat loss. Following Apgar scoring and a cursory physical assessment, the newborn may be weighed and measured (length, head, and chest circumferences). Aquamephyton (vitamin K) may be administered intramuscularly at this time. Positive identification of mother and baby may be established with matching bands, newborn footprints and/or mother's fingerprint. If the condition of the newborn is stable, he may be bundled and held by his father until physical care of the mother is complete.

A woman who plans to breastfeed may have the opportunity to nurse her baby soon after delivery. The newborn is usually alert for about one hour after birth. His vision is thought to be within an eight-inch field. Encouraging mother-father-baby interraction at this time is important.

TABLE 1-2   Apgar Score Chart*

OBSERVATION	SCORE		
	0	1	2
Heart Rate	Absent	Slow (below 100)	Over 100
Respiratory effort	Absent (apneic)	Slow, irregular, shallow	Good, sustained cry; regular respirations
Reflex irritability	No response	Grimace, frown	Sneeze, cough, cry
Muscle tone	Limp, completely flaccid	Some flexion of extremities; some resistance to extension of extremities	Active motion, good muscle tone, spontaneous flexion
Color	Cyanotic, pale	Body pink, extremities blue	Completely pink

*From: Apgar, V: *A proposal for a new method of evaluation of the newborn infant.* Curr Res Anesth Analg 260–267, 1953, with permission.

A one percent (1%) solution of silver nitrate ($AgNO_3$) is the most frequently used eye prophylactic for gonococcal infection (ophthalmia neonatorum), a potentially blinding disease of the conjunctiva. The Committee on Ophthalmia Neonatorum of the National Society to Prevent Blindness recommends the following:[4]

1. Eye prophylaxis for all newborns should be given within *one hour* after birth. Although $AgNO_3$ is most commonly used, Erythromycin (0.5%) or Tetracycline (1%) ophthalmic ointment or drops are considered equally effective.

2. The eyelids and surrounding skin of the newborn should be carefully cleaned with sterile cotton balls.

3. Two (2) drops of $AgNO_3$ should be instilled into both eyes (o.u.), manipulating the lid to insure that all parts of the conjunctival surface are reached.

4. DO NOT IRRIGATE THE EYES. Excess $AgNO_3$ may be gently wiped off after one minute.

Although eye treatment is a legal requirement governed by state law for all newborns, the instillation of eye drops may be safely delayed for one hour after birth. The nurse should try to delay the newborn's eye treatment within the safe time period to prevent clouding of vision during the first hour of life and perhaps facilitate maternal attachment. A recent study[5] indicated that early administration of $AgNO_3$ decreases eye openness in the newborn. Maternal response to the newborn's decreased visual responsiveness was of no consequence, that is, the mother's pleasure and excitement during the first hour after birth was not altered. It was hypothesized that newborn eye openness may encourage more affectionate attention from the father.

Emergency Delivery—A Nursing Responsibility

Occasionally, a woman's labor may progress more rapidly than expected. The nurse may find herself in the position of having to assist with the delivery of the baby. This can occur either outside the hospital setting or within the hospital before the doctor arrives. Regardless of the setting, the patient will usually experience a sense of panic about the imminent delivery. When a woman shouts, "The baby's coming!" speed is essential. The nurse should *first observe the perineum* to determine how much preparation time she has. While helping the woman to assume a comfortable position, it is essential to decrease her panic. Short positive verbal commands are best. Using a calm voice the nurse must convey an understanding of the woman's fears and the intention to help make this as safe and positive an experience as possible. Encourage the woman to pant during each contraction to decrease the urge to push (see Chapter 8). It may be necessary to pant with her.

If time permits, the nurse should wash her hands thoroughly. Sterile gloves and drapes are available in the hospital setting. Outside the hospital, clean sheets, blankets, towels, clothing, or unread newspapers may be used to provide a clean surface.

As the woman pants through her contractions the nurse may facilitate stretching of the perineum with warm compresses and/or gently massaging the perineal tissue with forefinger (inside the posterior vaginal wall) and thumb (directly on the perineum). As the head begins to emerge the woman will need constant support and reassurance. The nurse should apply gentle pressure to the fetal head to facilitate slow delivery. She should never attempt to delay delivery with forceful pressure on the fetal head or by having the woman hold her legs tightly together. Delivery of the head should be slow and controlled. It is best achieved in between contractions, while supporting the perineum. Rapid delivery of the head may cause maternal perineal tears and fetal subdural or dural tears.

The fetal cord may be wrapped around the neck (nuchal cord). To check for this before the shoulders are delivered, the nurse slides 1 or 2 fingers between the back of the baby's head and the vaginal wall. If one or two loops exist it may be pulled out and slipped over the baby's head. If the loop is too tight the cord should be clamped in two places, cut between the clamps, and then unwrapped from the baby's neck.

Following delivery of the head, the mouth and nose are suctioned with a bulb syringe to remove fluid, mucus, and blood or wiped out with a clean cloth or finger. To deliver the shoulders, the nurse places her hands on both sides of the baby's head and exerts gentle downward pressure to deliver the anterior shoulder from under the symphysis pubis. Upward pressure will deliver the posterior shoulder next. The nurse then encourages the mother to bear down for delivery of the rest of the baby.

The baby is held at the level of the uterus for clamping and cutting the cord. The clamps are placed approximately 4 to 6 inches from the abdomen, and the cord is cut between the two clamps. Outside the hospital setting, clean shoe laces or strong cord may be used for clamping (do not use wire). It is not necessary to cut the cord if transport to a hospital is possible. If the cord must be cut, a sterilized razor, knife, or scissors is recommended. Placing the baby on the mother's abdomen or allowing the newborn to nurse at the mother's breast will facilitate contraction of the uterus, enhancing separation of the placenta. Following spontaneous expulsion of the placenta, if the cord has not been cut, the placenta may be wrapped in clean newspaper and wrapped with the baby. The placenta will provide warmth if the shiny side is placed against the baby and they are wrapped together. Care should be taken to avoid any tension on the cord if it is still attached to the baby.

If the newborn does not breathe spontaneously following suctioning, the baby should be placed in a head down position. Gently rubbing the baby's back or flicking the soles of the feet may be sufficient to initiate respirations. If respirations still do not occur, mouth-to-mouth resuscitation should be started.

Prevention of heat loss is important. The baby should be thoroughly dried as soon as possible. Placing him directly against the mother's skin and covering both mother and baby should be sufficient.

The nurse needs to write down important information such as the time of delivery; Apgar scores at one and five minutes; the time of placental expulsion and its condition; presence of a nuchal cord; color of amniotic fluid; and mother's blood type and Rh if known. Mother and baby should be positively identified before transporting to a hospital. Identification bands (tape or strips of cloth) should include mother's name, time of delivery, and sex of the infant.

Maternal safety is maintained by promoting uterine contractions to decrease blood loss following delivery of the placenta. Allowing the baby to nurse will stimulate the release of oxytocin, which causes the uterus to contract. If nursing is not possible, gentle fundal massage should be continued until the uterus becomes firm. However, caution should be used, since overstimulation of the uterine muscles may also lead to relaxation with resultant hemorrhage. Mother and baby should be transported to the nearest hospital as soon as possible for further evaluation and care.

Labor and delivery can be an exciting and meaningful experience. The nurse is the key person in providing permission, direction, and support for the expectant couple. Sensitivity to the couple's needs and provision for expression of individual desires can decrease feelings of helplessness and enhance feelings of control. Encouraging mother and father to explore their new baby can foster the bonds of attachment and influence life-long relationships.

Review Questions

1. Provide the appropriate Apgar score for each of the following:
    a. _____ heart rate: absent
    b. _____ muscle tone: active motion
    c. _____ reflex irritability: grimace
    d. _____ respiratory effort: slow—irregular
    e. _____ color: completely pink

2. There is a direct correlation between the five-minute Apgar score and newborn:

a. mortality   c. development
b. growth   d. mental ability

3. The most frequently used prophylactic for gonococcal infection of the conjunctiva is a one percent solution of _____ .

4. When a woman in labor shouts "The baby's coming!" the first action by the nurse should be to:
   a. control the woman's panic
   b. observe the perineum
   c. call the doctor
   d. wash her hands

5. Warm compresses and/or gently massaging the perineal tissue just prior to delivery will facilitate perineal _____ .

6. Which of the following is the most appropriate method of safely promoting slow delivery of the fetal head?
   a. applying gentle pressure to the fetal head
   b. tightly crossing the woman's legs
   c. applying forceful pressure to the fetal head
   d. encouraging the woman to push with her contractions

7. The umbilical cord wrapped around the fetal neck is called a _____ cord.

8. Prior to clamping the umbilical cord, the newborn should be placed:
   a. on the mother's abdomen
   b. at the level of the uterus
   c. below the level of the uterus
   d. in a head down position on the mother's abdomen

Answers

1. The appropriate Apgar score for each of the following is:
   a. __0__ heart rate: absent
   b. __2__ muscle tone: active motion
   c. __1__ reflex irritability: grimace
   d. __1__ respiratory effort: slow—irregular
   e. __2__ color: completely pink
2. __a__ There is a direct correlation between the five-minute Apgar score and newborn mortality.
3. A one percent solution of *silver nitrate (AgNO₃)* is most frequently used prophylactically for gonococcal infection of the conjunctiva.
4. __b__ When a woman in labor shouts "The baby's coming!" the first action by the nurse should be to observe the perineum.

5.   Warm compresses and/or gently massaging the perineal tissue just prior to delivery will facilitate perineal *stretching*.
6.   <u>a</u>   The most appropriate method of safely promoting slow delivery of the fetal head is by applying gentle pressure to the fetal head.
7.   The umbilical cord wrapped around the fetal neck is called a *nuchal cord*.
8.   <u>b</u>   Prior to clamping the umbilical cord, the newborn should be held at the level of the uterus.

REFERENCES

1.   LIGGINS, CC: *Fetal influences on myometrial contractility.* Clin Obstet Gynecol 16:148, 1973.
2.   OXORN, H AND FOOTE, WR (deceased): *Human Labor and Birth,* ed 4. Appleton-Century-Crofts, New York, 1980, p 547.
3.   LEDERMAN, RP: *Evaluating uterine contractions.* In MALINOWSKI, JS, ET AL (EDS): *Nursing Care of the Labor Patient.* FA Davis, Philadelphia, 1978, p 13.
4.   National Society to Prevent Blindness: *Prevention and Treatment of Ophthalmia Neonatorum.* Revised 4/81.
5.   BUTTERFIELD, PM, ET AL: *Does the early application of silver nitrate impair maternal attachment?* Pediatrics 67(5):738, 1981.

BIBLIOGRAPHY

American Academy of Pediatrics: *Care of the Newborn in the Delivery Room.* Pediatrics 64(6):970, 1979.
BASH, DB AND GOLD, WA: *The Nurse and the Childbearing Family.* John Wiley & Sons, New York, 1981.
BOWE, NL: *Intact perineum: A slow delivery of the head does not adversely affect the outcome of the newborn.* J Nurse-Midwifery 26(2):5, 1981.
BUTTERFIELD, PM, ET AL: *Does the early application of silver nitrate impair maternal attachment?* Pediatrics 67(5):737, 1981.
CARR, KC: *Obstetric practices which protect against neonatal morbidity: Focus on maternal position in labor and birth.* Birth and Family Journal 7(4):249, 1980.
CLARK, AL, ET AL: *Childbearing: A Nursing Perspective,* ed. 2. FA Davis, Philadelphia, 1979.
DIONNE, KE: *If you must deliver a newborn.* RN 44(9):36, 1981.
HAWKINS, JW AND HIGGINS, LP: *Maternity and Gynecological Nursing.* JB Lippincott, Philadelphia, 1981.
JENSEN, MD, ET AL: *Maternity Care: The Nurse and the Family,* ed. 2. CV Mosby, St. Louis, 1981.

KLAUS, MH AND KENNEL, JH: *Maternal-Infant Bonding.* CV Mosby, St. Louis, 1982.

LEDERMAN, E, ET AL: *Maternal psychological and physiologic correlates of fetal-newborn health status.* Am J Obstet Gynecol 139(8):956, 1981.

MALINOWSKI, J: *Bladder assessment in the postpartum patient.* J Obstet Gynecol Neonatal Nurs 7(4):14, 1978.

MCKAY, SR: *Maternal position during labor and birth: A reassessment.* J Obstet Gynecol Neonatal Nurs 9(5):288, 1980.

OCHLER, JM: *Family-Centered Neonatal Nursing Care.* JB Lippincott, Philadelphia, 1981.

OLDS, SB, ET AL: *Obstetric Nursing.* Addison-Wesley, California, 1980.

OXORN, H AND FOOTE, WR (deceased): *Human Labor and Birth,* ed 4. Appleton-Century-Crofts, New York, 1980.

PHILLIPS, CR AND ANZALONE, JT: *Fathering: Participation in Labor and Birth.* CV Mosby, St. Louis, 1978.

PILLITTERI, A: *Maternal-Newborn Nursing Care of the Growing Family,* ed 2. Little, Brown & Co, Boston, 1981.

READ, JA, ET AL: *Randomized trial of ambulation versus oxytocin for labor enhancement: A preliminary report.* Am J Obstet Gynecol 139(6):669, 1981.

SAIGAL, S, ET AL: *Observations on the behavioral state of newborn infants during the first hour of life. A comparison of infants delivered by the Leboyer and conventional methods.* Am J Obstet Gynecol 139(6):715, 1981.

SOSA, R, ET AL: *The effect of a supportive companion on perinatal problems, length of labor, and mother-infant interraction.* N Engl J Med 303:597, 1980.

Standards for Obstetrics, Gynecologic, and Neonatal Nursing, ed. 2. The Nurse's Association of the American College of Obstetricians and Gynecologists, 1981.

WIGGINS, JD: *Childbearing: Physiology, Experiences, Needs.* CV Mosby, St. Louis, 1979.

YAO, AC AND LIND, J: *Cord clamping time influence on the newborn.* Birth and Family J 4(3):91, 1977.

Post-Test

1. Match column I with column II

Column I	Column II
a. Progesterone Deprivation Theory	(1) _____ increased levels of prostaglandins stimulate uterine smooth muscle contractions
b. Oxytocin Stimulation Theory	
c. Uterine Stretch Theory	
d. Placental Degeneration Theory	(2) _____ pressure on nerve endings from the overdistended uterus causes
e. Estrogen Stimulation Theory	

f. Fetal Membrane-Arachidonic Acid-Prostaglandin Theory
g. Fetal Cortisol Theory

increased uterine irritability with subsequent contractions

(3) _____ increased protein, myometrial hypertrophy, and ATP promote the onset of labor

(4) _____ uterine contractions are caused by oxytocin from the anterior pituitary gland

(5) _____ decreased circulation and oxygenation of the placenta may initiate the onset of labor

(6) _____ labor may occur with the administration of cortisol and ACTH

(7) _____ uterine contraction activity increases as progesterone production decreases near term, initiating labor.

2. Identify the premonitory signs of labor using a check (✓).

_____ a. engagement in the primigravida
_____ b. flexion
_____ c. placenta previa
_____ d. internal rotation
_____ e. extension
_____ f. bloody show
_____ g. SROM
_____ h. increased backache

_____ i. − 3 station
_____ j. increased vaginal secretions
_____ k. occiput posterior position
_____ l. loose stools
_____ m. 2–3 pound weight loss
_____ n. hydramnios

3. The settling of the uterus and its contents into the pelvis is called

_____ .

4. The passage of the largest diameter of the fetal presenting part into the maternal pelvic inlet is called _____ .

5. Match column I with column II.

Column I	Column II
a. true labor	(1) _____ Walking decreases the discomfort of contractions.
b. false labor	(2) _____ Contractions do not increase in frequency, intensity, or duration.

(3) _____ Contractions progressively increase in frequency and duration.

(4) _____ Contractions do not cause cervical dilatation.

(5) _____ Walking usually intensifies contractions.

(6) _____ Progressive cervical changes occur.

6. Gradual thinning of the internal cervical os is called _____ _____ .

7. Gradual opening of the cervix to 10 cm is called _____ _____ .

8. Vaginal discharge that occurs prior to or during labor and is thick, mucousy, and pink or dark red is called _____ .

9. Abnormal implantation of the placenta in the lower uterine segment is called _____ _____ . If the placenta covers the cervical os, the condition is classified as _____ . If it covers only a portion of the cervical os, it is classified as _____ .

10. A normally implanted placenta that separates from the uterine wall prior to delivery of the baby is called _____ _____ .

11. Use a check (✓) to identify the following normal characteristics of amniotic fluid when the fetus is in a vertex presentation.

_____ a. clear or cloudy   _____ e. strong odor
_____ b. meconium stained   _____ f. 1000 ml
_____ c. pale yellow   _____ g. greater than 2000–
_____ d. greenish color   3000 ml

12. The presence of meconium may be considered normal in which of the following presentations?

a. vertex   c. occipital
b. breech   d. cephalic

13. Excessive amniotic fluid is often associated with fetal malformations in which the fetus is unable to swallow and urinate normally in utero. This is called _____ or _____ .

14. Use a check (✓) to identify which of the following tests are used to establish the presence of amniotic fluid obtained from the vaginal vault.

_____ a. nitrazine test tape   _____ d. cervical mucus
_____ b. amniotomy   ferning
_____ c. fetal fat cell staining   _____ e. ultrasound
                                                _____ f. vaginal examination

15. Identify the appropriate stage of labor for each of the following (I, II, III, IV):

_____ a. the placental stage
_____ b. ends with complete dilatation
_____ c. 1 to 4 hours after delivery of the placenta
_____ d. begins with regular contractions
_____ e. fundal and lochia assessments are performed every 15 minutes
_____ f. average length of time for the primigravida is 12½–14 hours
_____ g. the stage of expulsion
_____ h. ends with delivery of the baby
_____ i. pushing is encouraged with contractions
_____ j. the period of greatest energy flow for the woman in labor
_____ k. signs of placental separation normally occur
_____ l. contractions bring about progressive dilatation and effacement of the cervix and descent of the fetus

16. Match column I with column II

Column I	Column II
a. Attitude	(1) _____ relationship between the presenting part of the fetus and the maternal pelvis
b. Lie	(2) _____ relationship of the longitudinal axis of the fetus to the longitudinal axis of the mother
c. Presentation	(3) _____ relationship of the fetal parts to each other—the degree of flexion or extension
d. Position	(4) _____ refers to the fetal part that is lowermost in the pelvis
e. Station	(5) _____ the level of descent of the presenting part in relation to the ischial spines of the maternal pelvis

17. Identify the appropriate landmark on the fetus that is used to determine position with each of the following:

Presenting Part	Presentation
a. occiput	(1) _____ face
b. forehead	(2) _____ frank breech
c. mentum	(3) _____ vertex
d. sacrum	(4) _____ complete breech
e. scapula	(5) _____ shoulder
	(6) _____ footling breech
	(7) _____ brow

18. Identify the mechanism of labor that each of the following statements describes:
    a. _____ The fetal head rotates from OT to OA (45 degrees), which places the occiput beneath the symphysis pubis.
    b. _____ The fetal head enters the pelvis OT.
    c. _____ Following delivery, the head rotates 45 degrees, placing the shoulders in the A-P diameter.
    d. _____ Resistance from the maternal pelvis forces the fetal head to present its smallest diameter.
    e. _____ Spontaneous delivery of the baby's body.
    f. _____ Delivery of the head occurs with this mechanism.
    g. _____ Immediate rotation of the fetal head (after delivery) 45 degrees back to the transverse position.

19. Mrs. Smith, a 20-year-old G-i, P-0 with a term pregnancy, is complaining of intermittent low back pain which has increased in frequency, duration, and intensity during the past 4 hours. Prior to admission to the labor area, which of the following might the nurse perform in assessing Mrs. Smith. Place a check (✓) in front of the appropriate actions.
    _____ a. Palpate contractions for frequency, duration, and intensity.
    _____ b. Obtain vital signs, including FHR.
    _____ c. Obtain an x-ray pelvimetry.
    _____ d. Perform Leopold's maneuvers.
    _____ e. Administer an enema and perineal prep.
    _____ f. Obtain a catheterized urine specimen.
    _____ g. Assess cervical dilatation and effacement via vaginal examination.

20. Leopold's maneuvers are used to manually determine fetal position and presentation. Identify the appropriate maneuver for each of the following (first, second, third, fourth):
    a. _____ The head is the presenting part felt over the pelvic inlet.
    b. _____ The buttocks are identifiable in the fundus.
    c. _____ The flexed fetal brow may be identified if engagement has not yet occurred.

d. _____ The fetal back is outlined and small parts are identified.

21. Solid foods are not recommended during labor because of decreased:
    a. renal retention
    b. gastrointestinal absorption
    c. use of routine enemas
    d. liver function

22. A full bladder during labor may:
    a. cause urinary incontinence
    b. interfere with labor progress
    c. be ignored, since it is not significant
    d. cause nausea and vomiting

23. Use a check (✓) to identify appropriate nursing measures that may be employed during labor to promote comfort.
    _____ a. reinforcement of learned coping patterns
    _____ b. support to maintain position during contractions
    _____ c. encouraging the supine position during contractions
    _____ d. forcing oral fluids to combat dry mouth
    _____ e. teaching conscious relaxation and pelvic rock
    _____ f. providing back rubs and counterpressure
    _____ g. encouraging continual ambulation

24. List three fears a woman in labor might have about herself and three fears she might have about her baby.
    a. Fears the woman might have about herself:
       (1) _____
       (2) _____
       (3) _____
    b. Fears the woman might have about her baby:
       (1) _____
       (2) _____
       (3) _____

25. Using the chart below, fill in the appropriate cervical dilatation progression and contraction frequency and duration for each phase of the first stage of labor.

	Dilatation	Frequency	Duration
Latent Phase			
Early Active Phase			
Transition			

26. During which phase of the first stage of labor (latent, early active, transition) is each of the following most likely to occur?

a. _____ Irritable, unwilling to be touched

b. _____ Strong urge to push or bear down

c. _____ Becomes doubtful of ability to control pain

d. _____ May not feel ready for labor

e. _____ May be afraid to be alone

f. _____ Open to instructions and directions

g. _____ Periods of amnesia occur between contractions

h. _____ Fatigue becomes evident

i. _____ Period when the woman needs the most support

27. List three signs of placental separation following delivery.

a. _____

b. _____

c. _____

28. Baby Smith has been evaluated by the nurse at one minute after birth. The following observations were noted: Heart rate—over 100; Respiratory effort—slow, irregular, shallow; Reflex irritability—grimace, frown; Muscle tone—some flexion of extremities, some resistance to extension of extremities; Color—body pink, extremities blue. Using the Apgar scoring method, provide the appropriate score for each of the five areas plus the sum of scores to determine Baby Smith's Apgar score at one minute after birth.

a. _____ Heart rate

b. _____ Respiratory effort

c. _____ Reflex irritability

d. _____ Muscle tone

e. _____ Color

f. _____ Total Apgar score at one minute after birth

29. Baby Smith's total Apgar score at one minute provides an index for nursing care. Which of the following is the most appropriate nursing intervention?

a. initiate resuscitative measures

b. prevent heat loss by bundling the baby securely

c. facilitate bonding with parents

d. weigh, measure, and apply $AgNO_3$ drops

30. Circle True or False and explain your answer:

a. T   F   The most frequently used prophylactic for gonococcal infection of the conjunctiva in the newborn is a one percent solution of silver sulfate.

b. T F The laboring woman who thinks the baby is coming is usually feeling pressure, which causes her to panic; therefore, the most appropriate nursing action is to help decrease her panic.

c. T F Warm compresses and/or gently massaging the perineal tissue just prior to delivery will facilitate perineal stretching.

d. T F The most appropriate method of safely promoting slow delivery of the head is to apply forceful pressure to the fetal head.

e. T F Immediately following delivery, but prior to clamping the cord, the newborn should be placed at the level of the uterus.

f. T F Following emergency delivery outside the hospital setting, the placenta should always be separated from the baby to prevent contamination.

Answers

1. (1)f (2) c (3) e (4) b (5) d (6) g (7) a
   (1) *Fetal Membrane-Arachidonic Acid-Prostaglandin Theory*—increased levels of prostaglandins stimulate uterine smooth muscle contractions.

(2)   *Uterine Stretch Theory*—pressure on nerve endings from the overdistended uterus causes increased uterine irritability with subsequent contractions.

(3)   *Estrogen Stimulation Theory*—increased protein, myometrial hypertrophy, and ATP promote the onset of labor.

(4)   *Oxytocin Stimulation Theory*—uterine contractions are caused by oxytocin from the anterior pituitary gland.

(5)   *Placental Degeneration Theory*—decreased circulation and oxygenation of the placenta may initiate the onset of labor.

(6)   *Fetal Cortisol Theory*—labor may occur with the administration of cortisol and ACTH.

(7)   *Progesterone Deprivation Theory*—uterine contraction activity increases as progesterone production decreases near term, initiating labor.

2.   a, f, g, h, j, l, m. The following are premonitory signs of labor: engagement, uterine contractions, bloody show, ROM, increased backache, increased vaginal secretions, loose stools, 2–3 pound weight loss.

3.   *Lightening* is the settling of the uterus and its contents into the pelvis.

4.   *Engagement* is the passage of the largest diameter of the fetal presenting part into the maternal pelvic inlet.

5.   (1) b (2) b (3) a (4) b (5) a (6) a. *True labor* is characterized by the following: contractions progressively increase in frequency and duration; walking usually intensifies contractions; progressive cervical changes occur. *False labor* is characterized by the following: walking decreases the discomfort of contractions; contractions do not increase in frequency, intensity, or duration; contractions do not cause cervical dilatation.

6.   *Effacement* is the gradual thinning of the internal cervical os.

7.   *Dilatation* is the gradual opening of the cervix to 10 cm.

8.   *Bloody show* is the vaginal discharge that occurs prior to or during labor. It is thick, mucousy, and pink or dark red in color.

9.   *Placenta previa* is the abnormal implantation of the placenta in the lower uterine segment. It may be classified as *total,* if the placenta completely covers the cervical os; or *partial,* if it covers only a portion of the cervical os.

10.   *Abruptio placentae* is the premature (prior to the birth of the baby) separation of a normally implanted placenta.

11.   a, c, f. Amniotic fluid should be clear or cloudy, pale yellow, and 1000 ml or less.

12.   b. Meconium may be considered normal in a *breech* presentation.

13.   *Hydramnios or polyhydramnios* is the presence of excessive amniotic fluid. It is often associated with fetal malformations in which the fetus is unable to swallow and urinate normally in utero.

14. a, c, d. The following tests are used to establish the presence of amniotic fluid in the vaginal vault: Nitrazine test tape; fetal fat cell staining; cervical mucus ferning.

15. a. III b. I c. IV d. I e. IV f. I g. II h. II i. II j. II K. III l. I. *Stage I* includes the following: ends with complete dilatation; begins with regular contractions; average length of time for the primigravida is 12½–14 hours; contractions bring about progressive dilatation and effacement of the cervix and descent of the fetus. *Stage II* includes the following: the stage of expulsion; ends with delivery of the baby; pushing is encouraged; the period of greatest energy flow for the woman in labor. *Stage III* includes: the placental stage; signs of placental separation normally occur. *Stage IV* includes the following: 1 to 4 hours after delivery of the placenta; fundal and lochia assessments are performed every 15 minutes.

16. (1)d (2) b (3) a (4) c (5) e.
    (1) *Position* — relationship between the presenting part of the fetus and the maternal pelvis.
    (2) *Lie* — relationship of the longitudinal axis of the fetus to the longitudinal axis of the mother.
    (3) *Attitude* — relationship of the fetal parts to each other — the degree of flexion or extension.
    (4) *Presentation* — refers to the fetal part that is lowermost in the pelvis.
    (5) *Station* — the level of descent of the presenting part in relation to the ischial spines of the maternal pelvis.

17. (1) c (2) d (3) a (4) d (5) e (6) d (7) b. The *occiput* is the presenting part in a *vertex* presentation. The *forehead* is the presenting part in a *brow* presentation. The *mentum* is the presenting part in a *face* presentation. The *sacrum* is the presenting part in *frank breech, complete breech,* and *footling breech* presentations. The *scapula* is the presenting part in a *shoulder* presentation.

18. The mechanisms of labor are:
    a. *Internal rotation* — the fetal head rotates from OT to OA (45 degrees) which places the occiput beneath the symphysis pubis.
    b. *Descent* — the fetal head enters the pelvis OT.
    c. *External rotation* — following delivery, the head rotates 45 degrees, placing the shoulders in the A-P diameter.
    d. *Flexion* — resistance from the maternal pelvis forces the fetal head to present its smallest diameter.
    e. *Expulsion* — spontaneous delivery of the baby's body.
    f. *Extension* — delivery of the head occurs with this mechanism.
    g. *Restitution* — immediate rotation of the fetal head (after delivery) 45 degrees back to the transverse position.

19. a, b, d, g. Nursing assessment prior to admission to the labor area might include: palpate contractions for frequency, duration, and

intensity; obtain vital signs, including FHR; perform Leopold's maneuvers; assess cervical dilatation and effacement via vaginal examination.

20. Leopold's maneuvers include:
    a. *Third* — the head is the presenting part felt over the pelvic inlet.
    b. *First* — the buttocks are identifiable in the fundus.
    c. *Fourth* — the flexed fetal brow may be identified if engagement has not yet occurred.
    d. *Second* — the fetal back is outlined and small parts are identified.

21. b. Solid foods are not recommended during labor because of decreased gastrointestinal absorption.

22. b. A full bladder during labor may interfere with labor progress.

23. a, b, e, f. Nursing measures that may promote comfort during labor are reinforcement of learned coping patterns; support to maintain position during contractions; teaching conscious relaxation and pelvic rock; providing back rubs and counterpressure.

24. a. Fears the woman might have about herself are fear of pain, long labor, abandonment, internal injury, losing self-esteem, embarrassment, and helplessness.
    b. Fears the woman might have about the baby are fear of survival, injury, deformity, how the baby will get out or that the baby won't come out.

25.

	Dilatation	Frequency	Duration
Latent Phase	1–3 cm	5–20 min	10–30 sec
Early Active Phase	4–7 cm	3–5 min	30–45 sec
Transition	8–10 cm	2–3 min	45–60 sec

26. Latent — d, f; Early Active — c, e, h; Transition — a, b, g, i. During the *latent phase* the following may occur: may not feel ready for labor; open to instructions and directions. During the *early active phase* the following may occur: becomes doubtful of ability to control pain; may be afraid to be alone; fatigue becomes evident. During the *transition phase* the following may occur: irritable, unwilling to be touched; strong urge to push or bear down; periods of amnesia

occur between contractions; period when the woman needs the most support.

27. The three signs of placental separation are: a, the uterus becomes more global in shape and rises in the abdomen; b, the cord visibly lengthens outside the vagina; and c, a trickle or gush of bright red blood exits the vagina.

28. Using the Apgar scoring method, the nurse would evaluate Baby Smith as follows:

    a. <u>2</u> Heart rate — over 100
    b. <u>1</u> Respiratory effort — slow, irregular, shallow
    c. <u>1</u> Reflex irritability — grimace
    d. <u>1</u> Muscle tone — some flexion of extremities; some resistance to extension of extremities
    e. <u>1</u> Color — body pink, extremities blue
    f. <u>6</u> Total Apgar score at one minute after birth.

29. <u>a</u>. Since Baby Smith's one-minute Apgar score is 6, the most appropriate intervention is initiation of resuscitative measures. A score of 3 to 6 means the baby is moderately depressed.

30. a. <u>F</u> The most frequently used prophylactic for gonococcal infection of the conjunctiva in the newborn is *not* a one percent solution of silver sulfate; it is a one percent solution of *silver nitrate*.

    b. <u>F</u> The woman in labor who thinks the baby is coming is usually feeling pressure, which causes her to panic; however, the most appropriate nursing intervention is to first observe the perineum for signs of imminent delivery.

    c. <u>T</u> Warm compresses and/or gentle massaging of the perineal tissue just prior to delivery will facilitate perineal stretching.

    d. <u>F</u> The most appropriate method of safely promoting slow delivery of the head is *not* by applying forceful pressure to the fetal head, which may cause damage. Slow delivery of the fetal head is best accomplished by applying gentle pressure to the fetal head.

    e. <u>T</u> Immediately following delivery, but prior to clamping the cord, the newborn should be placed at the level of the uterus. This prevents a loss of blood to the placenta when held above the uterus, or an increased amount of blood from the placenta to the newborn when held below the level of the uterus.

CHAPTER 2

ASSESSING UTERINE ACTIVITY AND FETAL RESPONSE

Janet S. Malinowski

Assessing uterine activity and fetal response is commonly termed *fetal monitoring*. It has two components: assessment of uterine contractions (UC) and assessment of fetal heart rate (FHR). It is the responsibility of the nurse to assess both UC and FHR at least every 30 minutes during Stage I and at least every 15 minutes during Stage II. This chapter addresses the current practices in fetal monitoring. Because of the rapidly changing technology in the field of fetal monitoring, even the experienced labor nurse needs review and periodic update.

OBJECTIVES

Upon completion of this chapter, the reader will be able to:

1. Identify the anatomic parts of the pregnant uterus at term.
2. Use the following terms correctly:
   For UC—fundal dominance, increment, acme, decrement, tonus, frequency, duration, intensity, rest interval, primary and secondary uterine dystocia, hypo- and hypertonic, tetanic, incoordinate, coupling.
   For FHR—baseline, brady- and tachycardia, variability, decelerations (early, late, variable), accelerations, funic and uterine souffles.
3. Assess UC and FHR using acceptable techniques.

continued on next page

4. Demonstrate awareness of the need for alternate methods of assessment, e.g., intermittent vs. continuous, external vs. internal monitoring.
5. Explain the rationale for the nursing interventions performed during the assessment process.
6. Evaluate UC and FHR differentiating normal from abnormal.
7. When monitoring UC and FHR, implement nursing interventions that demonstrate sound nursing judgment and promote patient comfort.
8. Document nursing care related to UC and FHR.
9. Explain the purposes of fetal blood sampling and the Oxytocin Challenge Test.
10. Summarize the nursing interventions involved in fetal blood sampling and the Oxytocin Challenge Test.

ANATOMY AND PHYSIOLOGY OF THE UTERUS DURING LABOR

Rhythmic contractions in the uterus signal the onset of Stage I of labor. The uterus is a muscular sac made up of 3 layers: (1) the *perimetrium*— the outer covering; (2) the *myometrium*—the thick muscular layer; and (3) the *endometrium*—the inner glandular, supportive tissue layer (Fig. 2-1). The myometrium is composed of 3 types of muscle fibers: (1) a longitudinal layer on the outside; (2) an interlacing pattern of muscle fibers and blood vessels in the middle; and (3) an inner layer of circular fibers. As the pregnant uterus contracts the longitudinal muscles straighten the fetus so one fetal pole (the buttocks) is at the top of the uterus, and the other (the head) presses on the bottom of the uterus.

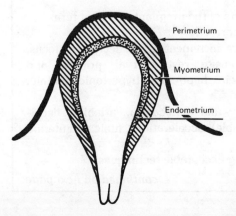

Perimetrium

Myometrium

Endometrium

Figure 2-1. Tissue layers of uterus.

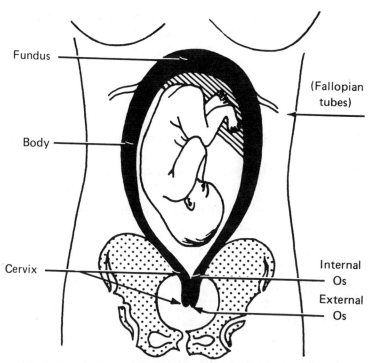

Figure 2-2. Anatomy of pregnant uterus at term.

Involuntary uterine contractions begin and are longest and strongest in the uppermost portion of the uterus, the *fundus*—therefore the term *fundal dominance*—and radiate downward over the *body* of the uterus (Fig. 2-2). With each UC the actively contracting muscles in the fundus shorten or retract, thinning (effacing) and expanding (dilating) the more passive lower portion, the *cervix*. Upon complete effacement (100 percent) of the *internal os* (Fig. 2-3) and dilatation (10 cm) of the *external os*, the

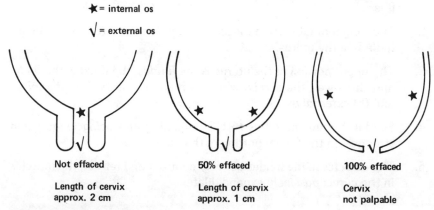

Figure 2-3. Cervical effacement.

cervix is no longer palpable and Stage II begins. It is then that the involuntary UC are supplemented by the voluntary forces of the abdominal and diaphragmatic muscles to expel the fetus through the birth canal.

Review Questions

1. Between the perimetrium and endometrium is the middle layer of the uterus called the _____ . It is composed of the following types of muscle fibers: a. _____ , b. _____ , and c. _____ .

2. A primary function of the longitudinal uterine muscles is to _____ _____ .

3. The upper portion of the uterus is called the _____ ____ , the middle portion the _____ , and the lower portion the _____ , which is made up of the a. _____ and b. _____ .

4. Fundal dominance refers to _____

5. Circle the correct term in the parentheses: The muscles in the fundus (actively, passively) contract and retract; the muscles in the cervix (actively, passively) expand/dilate.

Answers

1. The middle layer of the uterus is called the *myometrium,* which is composed of a. *longitudinal,* b. *interlacing,* and c. *circular* muscle fibers.

2. The longitudinal uterine muscles straighten the fetus so it is longitudinal in the uterus.

3. The upper portion of the uterus is the *fundus,* the middle, the *body,* and the lower, the *cervix,* which is made up of the (a) *internal os* and (b) *external os.*

4. Fundal dominance refers to UC beginning and being longest and strongest in the fundal portion of the uterus.

5. The muscles in the fundus *actively* contract and retract; the muscles in the cervix *passively* expand/dilate.

Terminology for Describing Uterine Contractions

UC have a characteristic pattern which is diagrammed in Figure 2-4. The *increment* is from the beginning of the UC until its peak strength. There is a gradual build up to this point, and the majority of the contraction time is involved in this portion. During early labor the actual onset of the UC may be difficult to determine. The *acme,* or peak, is the period of greatest uterine contractility—50 to >100 mm Hg of intrauterine pressure. The *decrement* is from the end of the acme until the termination of the contraction. Between contractions the uterus normally assumes a resting tone *(tonus),* ranging from 5 to 15 mm Hg. Uteroplacental circulation, which is compromised during the contraction, is restored during this resting phase.

When describing the UC, the *frequency* is the time in minutes from the onset of one UC (beginning of the increment) until the onset of the next UC. Rarely do UC occur at exactly the same frequency (e.g., every 3 minutes), so several UC need to be timed and compared. At the onset of labor UC may be every 10 to 20 minutes, but typically the frequency becomes every 2 to 3 minutes during good labor. The *duration* is the time in seconds between the onset of the increment until the completion of the decrement—that is, from the beginning until the end of one contraction. In early labor the duration may be 15 to 20 seconds, but it eventually becomes approximately 60. The *intensity* is the strength of the contraction at the acme. The intensity can be: (1) compared with the degree of indentation, for example, mild like a soft nose, moderate like the somewhat resisting chin, strong like the nonindentable forehead; or (2) measured in millimeters of Hg (mm Hg) via an internal uterine catheter. The normal *rest interval* (relaxation period) between the end of one UC and the beginning of the next is at least 30 to 60 seconds.

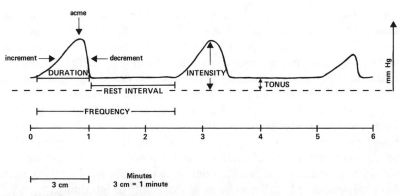

Figure 2-4. Pattern of uterine contractions.

Review Questions

Fill in the blanks with the correct terms:

1. From the beginning of the UC until its peak is the _____ _____.

2. The peak of the UC is the _____ .

3. From the peak to the end of the UC is the _____ .

4. The resting tone of the uterus is its _____ .

5. The period of time from the beginning of one contraction to the beginning of the next is the UC _____ .

6. The period of time from the beginning of one contraction to its end is its _____ .

7. By indenting the fundus during the peak of a contraction or noting the pressure displayed in mm of Hg via an internal monitor the UC _____ is determined.

8. The interval between the end of one UC and the beginning of the next is the _____ .

Answers

The correct terms are: (1) increment; (2) acme; (3) decrement; (4) tonus; (5) frequency; (6) duration; (7) intensity; (8) rest interval.

Uterine Contraction Assessment Methods

There are three ways to assess uterine contractions. The woman in labor usually provides a *subjective description*. It may be vague or detailed. It usually includes where the pressure is felt—in the back, in the suprapubic area, or beginning in the lower back and radiating around the abdomen. An objective assessment is done by the nurse or doctor by light fingertip *palpation of the fundus*. Care must be taken to differentiate between the uterine wall and adipose tissue. Palpation between contractions provides a basis for normal uterine tonus. With a contraction, gradual tensing and upward movement of the fundus can be felt and the frequency, duration, and intensity determined. As the woman nears Stage II, she may be irritated by palpation. *Electronic monitoring* provides an objective continuous assessment of UC. It can be done externally or internally.

For *external* monitoring of UC a transducer (also called tocotransducer or tocodynamometer) with a sensing button next to the abdomen is positioned over the greatest fundal surface. The transducer is held in place by an elastic strap that fits snugly around the abdomen. (No conductive paste or gel is necessary, since this is a sensor, not a conductor. When the transducer is cleaned, soapy water is used, not alcohol, which would remove the adhesive glue.) A rubber coated lead wire is attached from the transducer to the electronic monitor which graphically records the frequency and duration of the contractions, as well as other movements such as coughing, vomiting, and fetal activity. In the presence of normal uterine activity this monitoring device can be removed intermittently; this is advisable so the bathroom rather than bedpan can be used. (Portable machines are in the developmental stage.) Periodically the belts need to be re-adjusted and the (possibly reddened) skin underneath massaged. When the monitor is in place, the mother is usually in a lateral (preferably left lateral) or semisitting position. Although the external electronic method of monitoring UC is reliable, it has a few disadvantages. (1) Upon movement by the mother, the transducer frequently requires repositioning; therefore, there is a tendency to discourage movement. (2) Accurate recording in an obese mother is difficult, because good contact cannot be made with the uterine wall.

For *internal* monitoring of UC the cervix must be at least 2 to 3 cm dilated and, in most places, the membranes ruptured. Using sterile technique, the physician places a fluid filled catheter through the vagina into the uterus between the presenting part of the fetus and the pelvic bones. The catheter is secured to the mother's leg and connected to the monitor. Every 2 to 3 hours or so the catheter may need to be flushed out with sterile water to remove substances (e.g., vernix, mucus, air bubbles) that might clog the catheter. For accurate readings, the distal end in utero and proximal end of the catheter attached to the monitor should be at the same elevation with the transducer vented to the atmosphere. This monitoring device provides more accuracy than the external method, since it is not affected by extraneous movements. The absence of abdominal belts provides less restrictions on the mother, although she is usually confined to bed. However, there is an increased risk of uterine infection and perforation. By comparing the recorded tonus with the pressure during the acme of a contraction, the internal monitor can be used to determine the UC intensity. An increase of approximately 25 mm is mild, 50 mm is moderate, and 70 or greater is strong intensity.

Review Questions

1.   When palpating UC where and how is it done?

_____

_____

_____

_____

2. What nursing interventions are necessary when an external monitor is used to assess UC?

_____

_____

_____

_____

3. What modifications in nursing care occur when an internal monitor replaces an external monitor?

_____

_____

_____

_____

Answers

1. When palpating UC:
   —use fingertips gently on the uterine fundus;
   —determine the tonus and rest interval between contractions;
   —determine the frequency between contractions, duration of each contraction, and intensity (by indenting at the acme).

2. When using an external UC monitor:
   —position, and reposition as necessary, the transducer over the greatest fundal surface;
   —secure the transducer with an elastic belt;
   —interpret the UC frequency and duration using the graphic recording;
   —palpate the UC acme to assess the intensity;
   —(usually) position the mother on her side;
   —discourage excessive movement by the mother;
   —provide skin care under the transducer and belt as necessary;
   —in the presence of normal uterine activity and no other complications, periodically remove the monitor device to permit ambulation to the bathroom.

3. Modifications in nursing care when an internal monitor replaces an external monitor include:
   —more movement is permitted;
   —UC intensity can be determined by the graphic recording rather than by palpation;
   —uterine catheter flushing may be necessary every 2 hours.

Abnormal Uterine Contraction Patterns

Several abnormalities in UC patterns may be identified by the nurse. (1) Normally contractions become more frequent, longer in duration, and stronger in intensity. *Primary uterine dystocia* exists when nonprogressive contractions persist from the onset of labor and result in no cervical changes. (The term inertia is not used here, because of its unclear meaning.) (2) Well-established efficient (i.e., causing cervical changes) contractions should not become weak or cease; if they do, *secondary uterine dystocia* exists. (3) In either primary or secondary uterine dystocia the presence of weak ineffective contractions is called *hypotonic contractions*. Labor will not progress with such contractions. (4) Conversely, contractions can be *hypertonic,* that is, excessive in frequency, duration, or intensity. Contractions of 90 seconds or more duration are *tetanic.* These contractions are painful and could cause uterine rupture if allowed to continue. (5) When contractions originate in the mid- or lower uterine segment (i.e., with no fundal dominance), they are *incoordinate;* evidence of such is seen in the lack of cervical dilatation despite painful contractions. (6) It is abnormal to have less than 30 seconds relaxation between the end of one contraction and the beginning of the next, as well as for the uterus to not return to a tonus of 15 mm Hg or less. Two consecutive contractions with little or no rest interval is termed *coupling.*

Review Questions

To demonstrate your correct use of the terms for abnormal uterine contraction patterns, place the letter of each term in front of its description:

DESCRIPTION	TERM
1. _____ Nonprogressive contractions from the onset of labor	a. coupling
	b. hypertonic contractions
	c. hypotonic contractions
2. _____ Well-established contractions become weak or cease	d. incoordinate contractions
	e. primary uterine dystocia
	f. secondary uterine dystocia
3. _____ Weak ineffective contractions	g. tetanic contractions
4. _____ Excessively intense, long contractions	
5. _____ Contractions lasting 90 seconds or more	

6. _____ Contractions that are not fundal dominant
7. _____ Consecutive contractions with little or no rest interval

Answers

(1) e; (2) f; (3) c; (4) b; (5) g; (6) d; (7) a.

It is the responsibility of the labor nurse to assess carefully and chart the uterine activity of a woman in labor. Included should be: (1) subjective and objective findings; (2) nursing measures taken to relieve discomfort from the monitoring methods; (3) use of a more precise assessment method in the presence of suspicious UC; and (4) reporting any abnormal findings to the doctor. Often UC become more effective if the anxiety level of the woman is decreased; sensitivity and responsiveness to the individual's needs may facilitate improved UC. The relaxation techniques discussed in Chapter 8 are usually very helpful.

METHODOLOGY FOR ASSESSING FETAL HEART RATE

UC are regarded as stressful to the fetus, because they intermittently decrease the oxygen supply from the uterus to the fetus. Normally the fetus has enough reserve to compensate; however, this is not always true. The FHR is significant because it is the chief means of measuring fetal well-being or fetal distress during labor. It is the nurse who is primarily responsible for assessing the rates and knowing when abnormal FHR occurs.

Intermittent FHR assessment is most meaningful if it is done during the contraction and continued for 30 seconds beyond the end of the contraction. Because the rate is rapid and assessment is often interrupted by environmental distractions (e.g., fetal movement), the counting of the FHR is done best in two or four 15-second segments. The rate is then figured for the beats per minute (BPM).

EXAMPLES:

Getting 30 and 32 for two 15-second segments, multiply 62 by 2 for BPM.

Getting 30, 32, 35, and 31 for four 15-second segments, add them together for BPM.

The FHR is most often heard loudest where the fetal back is closest to the mother's abdomen. If the rate is not clearly audible, reposition the assessment apparatus. *Funic souffle,* a soft blowing sound created by the blood flowing through the umbilical vessels, should not be confused with FHR sounds, although the rate is the same.

Review Questions

1. In relation to a UC, when is the best time to assess the FHR?
   _____

2. What counting technique is recommended for determining the FHR?
   _____

3. Over what fetal part is the FHR most audible? _____

4. What is the term for the soft blowing sound that occurs as blood flows through the umbilical vessels? _____

Answers

1. The best time to assess the FHR is during the UC and within 30 seconds of the end of the UC.
2. The recommended technique for counting FHR is to count in 15-second segments, obtain at least two 15-second segments, and determine BPM.
3. The FHR is heard best over the *fetal back*.
4. *Funic souffle* is the term for the soft blowing sound that occurs as blood flows through the umbilical vessels.

Apparatus Used to Assess FHR Intermittently

Several apparatus can be used for intermittent FHR assessment. A *stethoscope* is the least effective. A *fetoscope* is a modified stethoscope with a head piece (Fig. 2-5A, B) that permits bone conduction from the listener's skull and therefore increases the audibility of the FHR. This inexpensive apparatus is convenient for FHR auscultation in normal situations; however, the woman should be in a supine position. A fetoscope is less accurate in detecting FHR changes during UC and through an obese abdomen. Only gross abnormalities of the FHR may be detected with a fetoscope. A Leffscope, or weighted fetoscope (see Fig. 2-5C), may be used in place of a fetoscope; it is especially useful when assessing FHR under sterile drapes used in the delivery room. A *Doppler unit* (e.g., Doptone, Fetone) is a portable rechargeable electronic instrument that amplifies the sound of the FHR (See Fig. 2-5D and E). With the volume turned down (to prevent

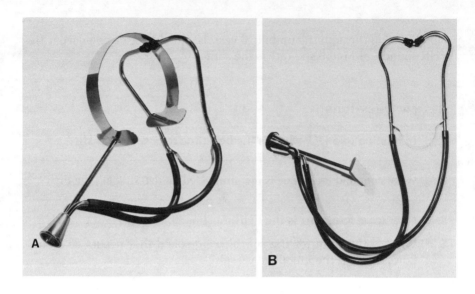

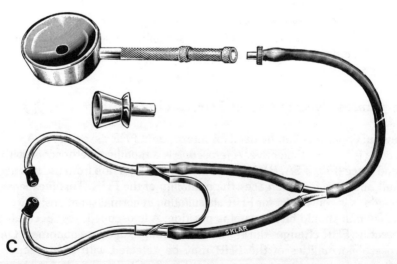

Figure 2-5. Fetoscopes. DeLee-Hillis stethoscopes: (A and B) head scope model, forehead rest model; (C) Leff stethoscope with weighted bells. (DeLee-Hillis photographs from: Graham-Field Surgical Company, Inc., New Hyde Park, NY 11040; Leff stethoscope photograph from: J. Sklar Manufacturing Company, Inc., Long Island City, NY 11101, with permission.)

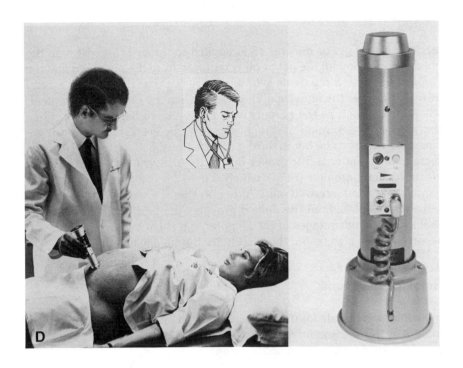

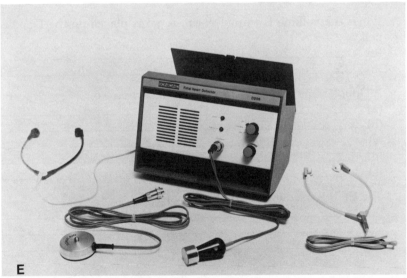

Figure 2-5. *(Continued).* (D and E) Grafco Mini Echo-Sounder and Sonicaid fetal heart detector. (Grafco Mini Echo-Sounder photograph from: Graham-Field Surgical Company, Inc., New Hyde Park, NY 11040; fetal heart detector photograph from: Sonicaid Medical, Inc., Fredericksburg, Va. 22404, with permission.)

static noise), a gel or mineral oil is applied to the bell to assist with the conduction of sound; the gel or oil is removed from the abdomen and the Doppler bell with a dry tissue following every use. The Doppler has several advantages over the fetoscope. It is useful when the FHR is hard to hear, when others such as the parents would also like to hear the rate, when the mother is assuming a sitting, side-lying or even standing position, when the rate is to be heard during contractions, and when FHR assessment is done under sterile drapes during the delivery. A more stationary *electronic fetal monitor* (EFM), which is used for continuous monitoring, can also be used intermittently. Although this is a very expensive apparatus, if it is already in the unit, it provides the best audio feedback as well as all the advantages of the Doppler; if it is left in place for 15 to 60 seconds, it will also record the FHR both graphically and digitally.

Review Questions

Indicate the rationale for the following nursing interventions during intermittent FHR assessment:

1. The fetoscope is worn on the head.

    _____
    _____
    _____

2. When the volume is turned down, a gel is placed on the Doppler bell.
    (a) _____
    (b) _____

3. A Doppler unit is used instead of the fetoscope.
    (a) _____
    (b) _____
    (c) _____
    (d) _____
    (e) _____

4. The EFM is used instead of the Doppler unit.

    _____
    _____
    _____

Answers

1. The fetoscope is worn on the head to permit bone conduction, thereby increasing audibility of the FHR.

2. When using a Doppler unit: (a) the volume is turned down when the gel is applied to prevent static noise; (b) the gel is applied to increase the FHR volume via conduction.

3. A Doppler unit is used instead of the fetoscope because (a) the FHR may be hard to hear with the fetoscope; (b) the parents may want to hear also; (c) the mother's position might be incompatible with use of the fetoscope; (d) the situation may indicate that the FHR should be heard during UC; and (e) sterile drapes on the mother may prohibit access to the abdomen.

4. The EFM may be used instead of the Doppler unit, because it provides better audio feedback and records both graphically and digitally if left in place for 15 to 60 seconds.

Continuous FHR Assessment

Continuous electronic fetal monitoring (EFM) provides a second-by-second audio and visual FHR recording (Fig. 2-6). Controversy exists among obstetricians regarding its routine use. There is little disagreement about its value in the high-risk obstetric patient, in the low-risk woman who develops problems during labor, and in the labor being augmented by oxytocin. Whether or not continuous monitoring is warranted in the uncomplicated low-risk woman is debatable.

Continuous EFM can be done externally or internally. In both cases the FHR is audible via a volume control knob. Depending on the brand of monitor the heart rate is heard as heart sounds or beeps. The volume should be adjusted so it is not disturbing to the mother and may be turned up at times of assessment only. Many mothers request that the volume remain audible so they can hear the baby during labor. The FHR is

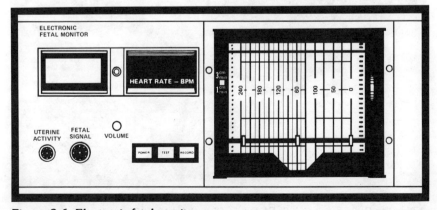

Figure 2-6. Electronic fetal monitor.

displayed digitally or on a circular disk as well as on a graph or printout (usually set to move 3 cm per minute), which becomes part of the woman's permanent chart. Because the monitor is very sensitive, the smallest variations in the FHR will be seen. The woman needs to be informed that 1 to 2 seconds of a comparatively low or high FHR are not signs of danger. When in doubt about the accuracy of the monitor's data, the actual FHR can be verified by auscultation with a fetoscope.

The *external EFM* has the advantage of being physiologically noninvasive. A lubricated ultrasound transducer is placed on the mother's (usually lower) abdomen over the site where the FHR is heard best. The transducer is secured by a snug abdominal strap (Fig. 2-7). (A similar tocotransducer and belt may be applied over the fundus to assess UC.) The distal end of the transducer is plugged into the monitor. Care must be taken that the monitor wire permits some movement of the mother.

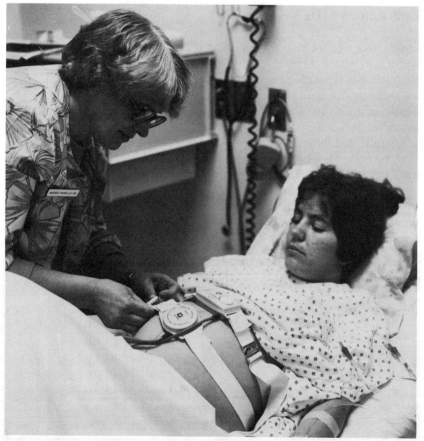

Figure 2-7. External monitor. (From: Clark, AL and Affonso, DD: *Childbearing: A Nursing Perspective*, ed. 2. FA Davis, Philadelphia, 1979, with permission.)

Occasionally the dried gel needs to be removed from the transducer and abdomen and reapplied to promote comfort as well as efficient ultrasound transmission. Readjustment of the transducer is necessary when heavily inked areas appear on the graph; such artifacts are due to mechanical problems in the monitor. In the presence of an accurate recording of a normal FHR the external EFM may be used throughout the labor. In the restless mother or very active fetus the external monitor may be ineffective. For the most precise assessment, internal monitoring is necessary.

An *internal EFM* can be applied once the membranes have ruptured, the cervix is dilated at least 2 to 3 cm, and the fetal presenting part can be reached. During a vaginal exam the doctor (or in some hospitals, the nurse) would insert an electrode through a guide about 1 mm into the fetal presenting part, avoiding the face, fontanels, and genitalia (Fig. 2-8). The guide tube surrounding the electrode and wires is removed, the color-coded wires are attached to the posts on the leg plate, electrode paste is applied, and the plate is strapped to the woman's leg. With the leads from the leg plugged into the monitor and the current on, precise variations in the FHR are recorded. Occasionally the electrode becomes dislodged from the fetus, especially during vaginal exams; at this time no FHR would be heard or recorded and re-application of the electrode would be necessary.

Although there is a slight risk of fetal infection at the site of the electrode insertion, the advantages of the internal monitor outweigh this disadvantage. Once in place it is more comfortable than the external

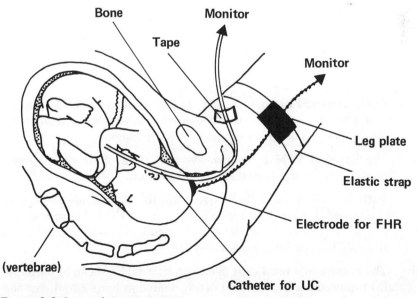

Figure 2-8. Internal monitoring.

monitor, allows for more movement by the mother, and provides a very accurate recording.

Review Questions

1. List three situations in which continuous EFM would more likely be used than intermittent EFM.
   a. _____
   b. _____
   c. _____

2. What advantage does the external EFM have over the internal EFM?
   _____

3. What nursing interventions are specific for the use of an external EFM?
   a. _____
   b. _____
   c. _____

4. What criteria must exist before an internal EFM can be applied?
   a. _____
   b. _____
   c. _____

5. Why would an internal EFM be used in place of an external EFM?
   a. _____
   b. _____

Answers

1. Continuous EFM would be used instead of intermittent EFM in: (a) high-risk obstetric patients; (b) low-risk women who have problems during labor; and (c) labors augmented by oxytocin.

2. The external EFM is noninvasive, therefore physically nontraumatic, and not a potential source of infection.

3. With the external EFM the nurse needs to: (a) lubricate and secure the transducer on the abdomen where the FHR is heard best; (b) provide for some movement despite lead wire; and (c) remove and re-apply the conductive gel as needed.

4. The criteria that must exist before an internal EFM can be used are: (a) ruptured membranes; (b) cervix dilated at least 2 to 3 cm; and (c) fetal presenting part can be reached.

TABLE 2-1　Clinically established FHR categories in BPM

< 100 = marked bradycardia
100–119 = moderate bradycardia
120–160 = normal
161–180 = moderate tachycardia
>180 = marked tachycardia

5.　The internal EFM will be used in place of an external EFM when: (a) there is a poor recording from the external EFM owing to mother's restlessness and/or fetal hyperactivity; and (b) a more precise assessment is needed than what the external monitor provides.

Determining the FHR Baseline

Each fetus has a unique FHR baseline level. By evaluating his FHR for a 10-minute period, it is possible to determine the range that exists for the major portion of the time. The range between UC is the *FHR baseline*. Normally the range is within 120 to 160 beats per minute (BPM). Table 2-1 identifies how FHR baselines beyond the normal range are classified. During the course of labor the baseline may change; a new baseline exists if the FHR remains within a new range for *longer than 10 minutes*.

EXAMPLE: Originally an FHR baseline may be 124 to 144 BPM (that is, normal). If the FHR rises to 160 to 170 BPM for longer than 10 minutes, it is relabeled moderate tachycardia; if it falls and remains below 120 for longer than 10 minutes, it is relabeled bradycardia.

The terms *tachycardia* and *bradycardia* refer specifically to baseline FHR. Tachycardia is often associated with a premature fetus, maternal fever, and minimal fetal oxygenation. The occurrence of tachycardia may be an early sign of fetal distress. Persistent bradycardia is found in a fetus with a congenital heart lesion. Occasionally the mother's heart rate may be mistakenly identified as the FHR. This muffled sound is called a *uterine souffle*. To avoid this error the mother's radial pulse should be felt simultaneously with listening to the FHR when fetal bradycardia is suspected.

Review Questions

1.　How is FHR baseline determined?

_____

_____

2.　What is the normal FHR baseline range? _____

3. a. An FHR range higher than normal is called _____ .
   b. List three causes of this abnormality:
      (1) _____
      (2) _____
      (3) _____

4. a. An FHR range lower than normal is called _____ .
   b. What is a plausible explanation for a range persistently lower than the normal range? _____ .

5. What is a uterine souffle and how does it compare with the fetal and maternal heart rates?

_____
_____
_____

Answers

1. The FHR baseline is the range that the FHR assumes between UC during the major portion of a 10-minute period.

2. The normal FHR baseline range is *120 to 160 BPM.*

3. *Tachycardia,* a range higher than the normal range for more than 10 minutes, might be due to prematurity, maternal fever, and fetal hypoxia.

4. *Bradycardia,* a lower than normal FHR range that persists, is found in fetuses with *congenital heart lesion.*

5. Uterine souffle is the mother's pulse heard through a uterine vessel; this rate is lower than the normal FHR.

Recognizing FHR Variability

The FHR baseline shows variability (fluctuations) if the fetus has normal neurologic function. Normally the baseline varies by 6 to 25 BPM (EXAMPLES: normal baseline of 120 to 125 or 136 to 160). No variability and minimal variability (Fig. 2-9) may be associated with a 20 to 30-minute fetal sleep state, or the more serious conditions of fetal prematurity, reaction to drugs, congenital anomalies, acidosis, and hypoxia. The significance of marked variability is currently not known. Decreased variability (less than 6 BPM) is an indicator of fetal distress. It is the nurse's responsibility to record FHR variability and to notify the attending physi-

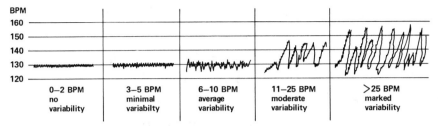

Figure 2-9. Fetal heart rate variability.

cian of deviations from normal. As stated earlier, the internal EFM is the most precise apparatus for determining variability.

Review Question

The normal variability of an FHR baseline is _____ BPM.

Answer

6 to 25 BPM is the normal variability.

Periodic Changes in the FHR

With each contraction there is a decrease in the blood flow in the inter-villous spaces in the placenta. The normal fetus has enough oxygen reserve that this decrease causes no apparent change in his FHR. But in some instances periodic changes occur in relation to UC. When the FHR falls below baseline level, and then returns, this is called a *deceleration*. If the FHR rises above the baseline, and then returns, this is called an *acceleration*.

Three types of decelerations have been identified: early, late, and variable (Fig. 2-10). *Early deceleration* is due to fetal head compression against the cervix. This causes an increase in intracranial pressure that initiates a vagal reflex, causing a temporary decrease in FHR. It is termed early because its onset is early in the UC. Its (uniform) shape reflects the intrauterine pressure curve, with the maximum amount of FHR deceleration consistently occurring at the acme of the contractions.

Late deceleration, an indication of fetal distress, is due to acute uteroplacental insufficiency resulting from a decreased blood flow during the UC. It is termed late, because its onset is late in the UC. Although its (uniform) shape also reflects the intrauterine pressure curve, it consistently occurs after the acme.

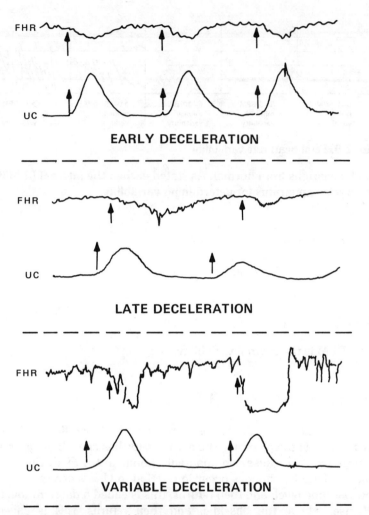

Figure 2-10. Types of fetal heart rate decelerations.

Variable deceleration, also an indication of fetal distress, is due to umbilical cord compression that decreases blood flow to the fetus at a variety of times. Therefore, the (variable) shape and onset of the deceleration do not correlate with the UC curve.

Review Questions

1. List the three FHR deceleration patterns and their causes.
    a. _____
    b. _____
    c. _____

2. Explain the rationale for the naming of each deceleration pattern.

_____

_____

3. Which two FHR deceleration patterns indicate fetal distress?

a. _____   b. _____

Answers

1. Early deceleration is due to fetal head compression. Late deceleration is due to acute uteroplacental insufficiency. Variable deceleration is due to umbilical cord compression.

2. The name of each deceleration pattern is based on the time of onset of deceleration in relationship to the UC.

3. Both late and variable deceleration indicate fetal distress.

No nursing intervention is necessary in the presence of early FHR decelerations, since this is an innocuous FHR pattern and has no apparent clinical significance; but intervention is necessary when late and variable FHR decelerations occur. The interventions are similar. (1) In order to increase the oxygen supply from the placenta through the umbilical cord to the fetus, the woman should be in a lateral position. If she lies on her left side, pressure is taken off the vena cava and therefore increases blood flow from the lower extremities. (Vena Cava Syndrome or Supine Hypotension Syndrome causes not only FHR deceleration but also maternal hypotension.) If the FHR does not increase because the cord is compressed while she is on the left side, then position on the right side should be assumed. If the FHR still does not increase, elevation of the legs or the Trendelenburg position may be necessary. (2) Severe UC may be the cause of inadequate fetal oxygenation. If oxytocin is infusing, it should be discontinued until further evaluation of fetal status occurs. (3) Oxygen via mask or nasal prongs may be given at 5 to 10 liters. (4) IV fluid should be given to increase the blood flow to the fetus. (5) The physician will need assistance if fetal blood sampling is performed.

Review Question

List five nursing interventions that would be appropriate in the presence of late or variable FHR deceleration.

a. _____

b. _____

c. _____

d. _____

e. _____

Answer

In the presence of late or variable FHR decelerations the woman's position should be altered to facilitate fetal oxygenation; infusion of oxytocin should be stopped; oxygen may be given; IV fluid should be started or the rate increased; and assistance should be given if fetal blood sampling is performed.

FHR *acceleration* is an increase in FHR at the time of the UC. It may have a shape that is *uniform* (similar) with the UC curve. The acceleration itself is not hazardous to the fetus but may be a very early indication of fetal compromise. Therefore, careful observation should be made for the occurrence of late decelerations if uniform accelerations exist. A *variable* acceleration (having little if any similarity in shape and relation to UC) is due to fetal movement; this is a sign of fetal well-being and is the primary focus of assessment in the nonstress test (refer to Chapter 6).

Review Question

What intervention should the nurse make in the presence of FHR accelerations?

_____

_____

_____

Answer

When FHR accelerations occur the nurse should observe the pattern of occurrence (that is, uniform and coordinated with UC); if such, watch further for late decelerations.

Although the EFM has made UC and FHR assessment more accurate and less time consuming it has one major drawback. Too often the monitor gets more attention than the human being it is attached to. It is not a substitute for skilled, individualized, supportive nursing care. The woman who is given a brief lesson about the EFM equipment and the information it provides often finds the monitor to be a source of reassurance. The nurse should get into the habit of always giving her primary attention to the woman in labor. The monitor is merely a technical tool that assists in the assessment process.

ASSESSING FETAL RESPONSE
BY FETAL BLOOD SAMPLING

Fetal hypoxia resulting in acidosis (a low pH, < 7.20) is suspected in the presence of an abnormal FHR pattern (late or variable decelerations, bradycardia or tachycardia, minimal variability). There is a good correlation between immediate newborn condition (that is, Apgar score) and fetal blood pH. An Apgar of greater than 7 (good condition) is usually consistent with a pH of greater than 7.25.

Since obtaining a fetal blood sample is done when there is a suspicion of fetal distress, the mother is likely to be anxious before the procedure even begins. The nurse, as the main source of emotional support, should stay with the mother and explain what is being done, since the doctor(s) will be absorbed in the technical aspects of the procedure. As the mother lies supine (or on her left side in the presence of supine hypotension syndrome), the mother's perineum is illuminated and cleansed and a cone-shaped instrument inserted vaginally through her cervix (membranes must be ruptured). A small light in the cone permits visualization of the fetal presenting part (scalp or buttocks), which is cleansed with a sterile swab, dabbed with silicone, and pricked with a blade. The blood is collected in a heparinized tube, and the tube is sealed, iced, and sent immediately to the lab for analysis. In order to decrease the incidence of fetal hemorrhage, pressure is placed on the puncture site through the next 2 UC—blood flows from the fetal scalp more freely during UC. Serial determinations (more than one sample) are necessary for reliable results. Continuous tissue pH monitoring is available but rarely used so far. In the presence of a borderline pH (7.20 to 7.25) another blood sample is taken within 15 to 30 minutes. Values of below 7.20 during Stage I and below 7.15 in Stage II usually result in termination of the labor by operative delivery (low forceps or cesarean).

Review Questions

1. Why is fetal pH sampling done? _____

2. What nursing interventions can be done to decrease maternal anxiety during the pH sampling procedure? _____

_____

3.   What would you expect to occur if the pH is < 7.20 with repeated samples? _____

Answers

1.   Fetal pH sampling is done *to determine the presence of fetal acidosis.*

2.   During this procedure the nurse can decrease maternal anxiety by *staying with the mother and explaining what is being done.*

3.   If < 7.20 pH is found in more than one sampling during Stage I, the woman would usually be *delivered immediately by low forceps or cesarean delivery.*

USING EFM IN THE OXYTOCIN CHALLENGE TEST

In antepartal situations in which a fetus is likely to be compromised owing to a low placental reserve (for example, postmaturity, low estriol excretion, toxemia, maternal diabetes, or hypertension), it is important to determine whether the fetus can tolerate the stress of UC. The Oxytocin Challenge Test (also referred to as OCT, Stress Test, Placental Sufficiency Test, and Fetal Reserve Test) causes physiologic stress by stimulating UC via oxytocin infusion.

Prior to the test the woman must sign a legal consent form and be forewarned that the procedure could stimulate labor. Before the test she is encouraged to eat a light meal (since food in the stomach decreases bowel sounds which otherwise interfere with the FHR recording) and to void (preventing interruption of the test). During the test her blood pressure is taken every 10 to 15 minutes to determine any changes that might affect the FHR. External uterine and fetal monitors are applied to the mother as she lies in a semi-Fowler position, tilted slightly to her left. The printout is observed for 10 to 30 minutes to determine the resting tone of the uterus and FHR baseline. In the presence of spontaneous UC activity every 3 minutes, oxytocin is not necessary.

Two tests for cord compression are performed before giving any oxytocin. (1) The Hillis maneuver involves exerting pressure on the fundus in the direction of the woman's feet. This presses the fetal chin against his chest. In the presence of a nuchal cord (cord around the neck), FHR variable decelerations result. (2) The Mueller maneuver involves putting suprapubic pressure on the fetal head. In the presence of a low-lying cord FHR variable decelerations result.

If no decelerations occur, oxytocin is given until the UC frequency is 3 within 10 minutes with a duration of 40 to 60 seconds. In the presence of late or variable decelerations, discontinue the oxytocin immediately; keep the primary IV infusing; have the mother lie on her left side; administer oxygen; and notify the physician immediately. See Chapter 6 for the interpretation of the test results.

Review Questions

1. Why is an OCT done?

2. Identify five preparatory measures that are done before giving the oxytocin in an OCT:
   a. _____
   b. _____
   c. _____
   d. _____
   e. _____

3. Why is the monitor used for 10 to 30 minutes before the oxytocin is started?

4. In the presence of no abnormal findings, what UC characteristics are desirable from the OCT?

Answers

1. OCT causes physiologic stress by stimulating UC. This test determines whether the fetus has enough placental reserve to tolerate the stress of UC.

2. Preparatory measures done before giving oxytocin in an OCT include:
   a. A consent form is signed.
   b. The woman is informed about the procedure, including the possibility of labor starting as a result.
   c. Consumption of a light meal is encouraged.
   d. The woman is instructed to empty her bladder.
   e. Her blood pressure is taken every 10 to 15 minutes throughout the test.

  f. External UC and fetal monitors are applied.

  g. The printout is observed for 10 to 30 minutes.

  h. Tests for cord compression are performed.

3. If spontaneous UC occur every 3 minutes on the printout, oxytocin is not necessary.

4. UC occurring 3 times in 10 minutes lasting 40 to 60 seconds are desirable during the OCT.

CONCLUSION

As this chapter indicates, assessment of UC and fetal response is not a simple procedure. Depending on the findings, assessment every 30 minutes during Stage I and every 15 minutes during Stage II may not be frequent enough. It is an area in which nurses are the primary assessors and in which nursing judgment and interventions are critical.

BIBLIOGRAPHY

BECK, CT: *Patient acceptance of fetal monitoring as a helpful tool.* J Obstet Gynecol Neonatal Nurs 9(6):350, 1980.

CRANSTON, CS: *Obstetrical nurses' attitudes toward fetal monitoring.* J Obstet Gynecol Neonatal Nurs 9(6):344, 1980.

DIAMOND, F: *High-risk pregnancy screening techniques.* J Obstet Gynecol Neonatal Nurs 7(6):15, 1978.

FRIEDMAN, EA: *Labor: Clinical Evaluation and Management,* ed 2. Appleton-Century-Crofts, New York, 1978.

GROSS, TL, SOKOL, RJ, AND ROSEN, MG: *Clinical use of the intrapartum-monitoring record.* Clin Obstet Gynecol 22(3):633, 1979.

HON, EH: *An Introduction to Fetal Heart Rate Monitoring,* ed 2. Corometrics Medical Systems, Inc., New Haven, 1975.

JENSEN, MD, BENSON, RC AND BOBAK, IM: *Maternity Care: The Nurse and the Family,* ed 2. CV Mosby, St. Louis, 1981.

KATZ, M, ET AL: *Neonatal heart rate reactivity following variable decelerations during labor.* Am J Obstet Gynecol 136(3):389, 1980.

KELLNER, KR, ET AL: *Evaluation of a continuous tissue pH monitor in the human fetus during labor.* Obstet Gynecol 55(4):523, 1980.

McDONOUGH, M, SHERIFF, D, AND ZEMMEL, P: *Parents' responses to fetal monitoring.* Am J Maternal Child Nurs 6(1):32, 1981.

NAACOG: *Standards for Obstetric, Gynecologic, and Neonatal Nursing,* ed 2. NAACOG, Washington, DC, 1981.

NAACOG: *The Nurse's Role in Electronic Fetal Monitoring.* NAACOG Technical Bulletin, #7, 1980.

OLDS, SB, ET AL: *Obstetric Nursing.* Addison-Wesley, Menlo Park, Calif, 1980.

OXORN, H: *Oxorn-Foote: Human Labor and Birth,* ed 4. Appleton-Century-Crofts, New York, 1980.

PILLAY, SK, ET AL: *Fetal monitoring: A guide to understanding the equipment.* Clin Obstet Gynecol 22(3):571, 1979.

POWELL, PW AND TOWELL, ME: *Abnormal fetal heart rate associated with congenital abnormalities.* Br J Obstet Gynaecol 87(4):270, 1980.

SETHI, S: *Oxytocin challenge test.* Am J Nurs 78:2112, 1978.

TUCKER, SM: *Fetal Monitoring and Fetal Assessment in High-Risk Pregnancy.* CV Mosby, St. Louis, 1978.

UMBECK, K AND DIAMOND, F: *An oxytocin challenge test protocol.* J Obstet Gynecol Neonatal Nurs 6(1):29, 1977.

WESTGREN, M, ET AL: *Intrapartum electronic fetal monitoring in low-risk pregnancies.* Obstet Gynecol 56(3):301, 1980.

ZIEGEL, E AND CRANLEY, M: *Obstetric Nursing,* ed 7. Macmillan, New York, 1978.

POST-TEST

1. Assessment of UC involves determination of activity in the uterine _____ , since this is where the activity is _____ . The parts of the UC include the following: the increasing intensity, called the _____ ; the strongest part, called the _____ ; and the decrease in intensity, called the _____ .

2. UC are described by the following three terms. Define them:
   a. frequency _____
   _____

   b. duration: _____
   _____

   c. intensity: _____

3. In the following situations, designate the correct term for the uterine activity:
   a. normally progressing UC become less frequent and less intense:
   _____

   b. UC 90 sec. duration or longer:
   _____

   c. normal uterine activity state between UC:
   _____

   d. UC that begin in the uterine body:
   _____

e. two consecutive UC that have less than 30 sec. relaxation between them: _____

f. uterine activity that from the start of labor continues to be weak and ineffective: _____

g. extremely forceful UC:

_____

h. weak ineffective UC: _____

4. Is it acceptable to:
   a. palpate the uterus between UC: _____Why?

   _____

   b. palpate the uterus throughout several UC? _____Why?

   _____

   c. base your assessment of UC on the mother's description? _____Why?

   _____

5. In the presence of which of the following situations would you consider using an external UC monitor instead of relying on intermittent assessment by palpation?
   a. during suspected primary or secondary uterine dystocia;
   b. during suspected tetanic UC;
   c. during suspected coupling of UC;
   d. during suspected hypotonic or hypertonic UC;
   e. during UC that are subjectively more painful to the mother than they objectively feel to the examiner?

6. What criteria must exist before an internal UC and/or FHR monitor can be applied?
   a. _____
   b. _____
   c. _____

7. Using A for fetoscope, B for Doppler unit or intermittent EFM, C for external EFM, and D for internal EFM, indicate which FHR assessment apparatus would be best to use in the following situations:
   a. _____ Early uncomplicated labor.
   b. _____ Oxytocin induction; membranes intact.
   c. _____ Normal FHR and UC; continuous graphing desirable.
   d. _____ Occasional variable decelerations following rupture of membranes.
   e. _____ On the delivery table with sterile drapes in place.

8. Use the correct term to describe each of the following FHR:
   a. baseline of 100 to 120 = _____
   b. periodic decrease with contractions = _____
      _____
   c. muffled sound consistent with maternal pulse but suspected to be FHR = _____

9.   Briefly chart and interpret the following patient data:
Situation A: Following 20 minutes on the external monitors, the FHR was seen to move frequently between 120 to 145, with a 1- to 2-second 160 BPM, when the mother felt the fetus move. Contractions were starting every 2 to 3 minutes and causing a slight decrease in FHR to 120 at the acme. The contractions were slightly indentable and were 40 to 50 seconds from beginning to end.

Your charting:

_____
_____
_____
_____
_____

Your interpretation:

_____
_____
_____
_____
_____

Situation B: The patient is rocking back and forth in bed, causing the monitors to trace poorly. She says the monitors bother her, and she wants them removed. Furthermore she is disturbed by the IV infusing oxytocin. Doctor Smith proceeds to replace the external monitors with internal EFM, using standard procedure, while the nurse explains the hows and whys. The monitor tracings give clear patterns with contractions starting every 1½ to 2 minutes, lasting 50 to 75 seconds — some with 20 seconds resting time — reaching 60 mm Hg pressure. FHR ranges from 130 to 134 between contractions with a consistent decrease to 115 beginning after the acme.

Your charting:

_____
_____
_____
_____

Your interpretation:

_____
_____
_____
_____

10. Explain why a woman who experienced a normal (negative) OCT might not be anxious when the physician begins induction with

oxytocin (including the use of monitors) but might be very anxious when fetal pH sampling is to be done.

_____

_____

_____

_____

_____

ANSWERS TO POST-TEST

1. Uterine activity is determined in the *fundus,* since this is where uterine activity is *dominant.* The increasing intensity is the *increment;* the strongest part is the *acme;* the decreasing intensity is the *decrement.*

2. Frequency is from the onset of one UC until the onset of the next. Duration is from the beginning until the end of the UC. Intensity is the strength of the UC at its acme.

3.   a.   *Secondary uterine dystocia* occurs when normally progressing UC become less frequent and less intense.
     b.   *Tetanic contractions* are of 90 seconds duration or longer.
     c.   *Tonus* (or the rested status) is the normal uterine activity state between contractions.
     d.   *Incoordinate contractions* are UC that begin in other than the fundus.
     e.   *Coupling* is two consecutive contractions that have less than 30 to 60 seconds relaxation between them.
     f.   *Primary uterine dystocia* is uterine activity that from the start of labor continues to be weak and ineffective.
     g.   *Hypertonic UC* are extremely forceful UC.
     h.   *Hypotonic UC* are weak, ineffective UC.

4.   a.   Palpation of the uterus between UC is acceptable to determine the degree and time interval of tonus.
     b.   Palpating the uterus throughout the UC is acceptable to determine the time of onset, the duration, the intensity (at the acme), and rest interval. This also gives a basis for comparing the UC for increase in frequency, duration, and intensity.
     c.   Basing your assessment of UC on the mother's description is not acceptable, since her interpretation is not objective.

5. In all of the situations (a–e) continuous assessment is necessary to verify if abnormal UC patterns exist. The external monitor provides a continuous measurement of the UC frequency and duration.

6. Before internal UC and/or FHR monitors can be applied, the cervix must be dilated 2 to 3 cm or more, the membranes must be ruptured, and the fetal presenting part must be reachable.
7. a. A — In early uncomplicated labor a fetoscope is used.
   b. C — When membranes are intact but continuous monitoring is needed because of the oxytocin induction, an external EFM is used.
   c. C — When continuous graphing is desirable and the FHR and UC are normal, external EFM is satisfactory.
   d. D — Occasional variable decelerations following rupture of membranes require an internal EFM if the criteria of cervical dilatation and reachable presenting part exist.
   e. B — On the delivery table when the sterile drapes are in place a Doppler unit is used (or possibly an external EFM).
8. Terms used to describe FHR include:
   a. A baseline of 100 to 120 is *bradycardia*.
   b. Periodic decrease with contractions is *deceleration*.
   c. A muffled sound in the FHR consistent with the maternal pulse is a *uterine souffle*.
9. SITUATION A.
   Charting: External EFM in place. FHR 120–145 baseline, accels with fetal activity, early decels noted. UC q 2–3½ mins., 40–60 sec., mod. intensity.
   Interpretation: All normal — baseline, healthy response from fetus, head compression with UC, UC that should eventually cause cervical changes.
   SITUATION B:
   Charting: Pt. restless. Requesting monitors' removal. Poor tracings. Dr. Smith applied int. EFM and uterine catheter using sterile technique. Procedure and purpose explained by nurse. Good tracings resulted. UC q 1½–2 min., some with 20 sec. of tonus, 50–75 sec. duration, 60 mm Hg intensity. FHR minimal variability 130–134 with late decels. to 115.
   Interpretation: Owing to patient's intolerance of external monitors and poor tracings, internal monitors were warranted (assuming criteria for such are met). Uterus was hyperactive with strong, too frequent UC and insufficient resting time between contractions. This resulted in uterine-placental insufficiency (late decels) which requires turning the mother to her left, discontinuing the oxytocin flow, and constantly monitoring UC and FHR. If late decels continue, the mother should be given oxygen and possibly placed in Trendelenburg or with legs elevated. Keep the doctor informed. Inform the mother of the reasons for these urgent interventions without increasing

her anxiety if possible. Cautious measures can be relaxed upon occurrence of q 2–3 minute or less frequent UC with resting interval of at least 30 sec. and FHR varying 6–25 BPM between 120–160 with no late or variable decels.

10. Both an OCT and oxytocin induction involve an IV (double set-up) with oxytocin, an infusion pump, and external FHR and UC monitors. The woman has experienced UC during the negative OCT. The equipment and initial procedures are very similar. Anxiety is likely when a fetal pH sampling is to be done, because not only is the procedure new to the woman but there are signs of fetal distress, which undoubtedly worry her.

CHAPTER 3

MECHANISMS OF LABOR: IMPLICATIONS FOR NURSING CARE

Janet S. Malinowski

This chapter presents the anatomy of the bony pelvis and its relationship to the normal movement of the fetus during the birth process. The chapter is divided into two parts: the normal mechanisms of labor through a gynecoid pelvis and nursing implications related to the mechanisms of labor.

Before beginning the first part, if the anatomic terms of the pelvis in Figure 3-1 are new to you, learn them before proceeding with this chapter.

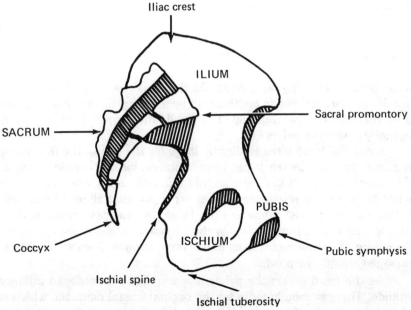

Figure 3-1. Anatomy of the bony pelvis.

OBJECTIVES

Upon completion of this chapter, the reader will be able to:

1. Briefly describe 3 adaptive processes that the fetal head must undergo as it moves through the maternal pelvis.
2. Identify the 7 mechanisms of labor in proper sequence, and the 3 pelvic planes.
3. Describe the passage of the fetus through the normal female pelvis.
    a. Identify the pelvic bones, the significant landmarks, and the normal female pelvic type.
    b. Identify the significant characteristics of each plane, pelvic diameters that are manually measurable, and the mechanisms as they occur in each plane.
4. Complete a pelvic measurements chart with the ideal findings for the normal mechanisms of labor to occur.
5. Use data that predict the occurrence of normal mechanisms of labor.
6. Apply 2 physical principles that influence fetal descent.
7. Explain 3 ways to promote changes in fetal position.

THE NORMAL MECHANISMS OF LABOR THROUGH A GYNECOID PELVIS

Adaptation by the Fetal Head

In the process of being born vaginally, the fetus passively adapts to the unyielding maternal pelvic architecture by molding, flexing, and rotating to fit through the passageway. The head, the largest fetal diameter, normally enters the pelvis first.

Since the head often is slightly large for the pelvis, the five bones that form the head, loosely joined by membranes, *mold* or override, thereby readjusting the head's diameter so that it fits into and through the bony pelvis despite some resistance. This is not to say that all fetal heads will fit through the pelvis. Some are too large. In that case cephalopelvic disproportion (CPD) exists. But in the presence of slight disproportion, given time, the head molds itself into a small enough diameter to permit passage through the pelvis.

As the head enters the pelvis it is usually in a nonflexed military attitude. There is usually room for the occipitofrontal diameter, which is 11.0 cm, to fit into the inlet of the pelvis (Fig. 3-2). As it moves through

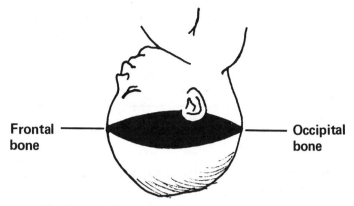

Figure 3-2. Occipitofrontal diameter.

the pelvis a smaller diameter is necessary. This is accomplished by *flexing* the neck, placing the chin on the chest. The result is a reduced diameter of 9.5 cm and is called the suboccipitobregmatic diameter—the area below the occipital bone moving around the head to the bregma (anterior fontanel) (Fig. 3-3).

Normally the fetal head enters the pelvis in an occiput transverse (OT) position. Upon meeting resistance it *rotates* 90 degrees to occiput anterior (OA) where the pelvic space is more accommodating.

Review Questions

Briefly describe the following adaptive processes that the fetal head goes through:

1. molding: _____

_____

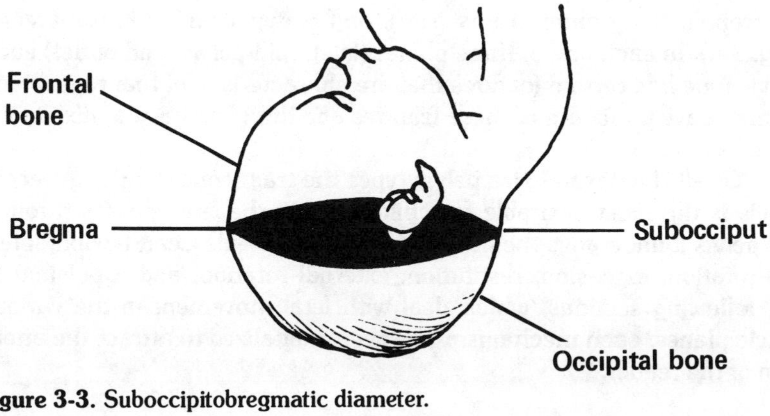

Frontal bone

Bregma ——————

Subocciput

Occipital bone

Figure 3-3. Suboccipitobregmatic diameter.

2. flexion: _____

_____

_____

3. rotation: _____

_____

_____

Answers

1. Molding: The bones in the fetal head readjust (mold), forming a smaller diameter.
2. Flexion: The fetal head normally enters the pelvis nonflexed with an 11 cm occipitofrontal diameter. By flexing the head it presents a 9.5 cm suboccipitobregmatic diameter.
3. Rotation: The fetal head rotates from OT to OA because that way it finds less resistance.

Pelvic Characteristics

The characteristics of the pelvis are usually assessed by the physician or nurse during the initial prenatal visit. The woman's obstetric record is likely to have a chart such as this:

PELVIC MEASUREMENTS: D.C. _____ , Spines _____ ,
Sacrum _____ , Arch _____ , Bitubs. _____ ,
Coccyx _____ , Type _____

It is recommended that the reader fill in the blanks on this chart, using the norms that are identified in italics in the succeeding sections.

Based essentially on the shape of the pelvic inlet, there are four basic pelvic types: gynecoid (normal female), android (normal male), anthropoid (long anterior-posterior), and platypelloid (wide transverse) (Fig. 3-4). In each one of three planes (inlet, mid-pelvis, and outlet) each pelvic type has certain features that are characteristic of that type. Many women have a mixture of these features and therefore have a mixed type of pelvis.

Of all the normal size pelvic types the true (consistently) gynecoid pelvis is the most desirable for childbirth. As the fetus passes through the pelvis it undergoes the mechanisms of labor—descent, flexion, internal rotation, extension, restitution, external rotation, and expulsion. In the following sections, which deal with fetal movement in the various pelvic planes, each mechanism has been capitalized to attract the attention of the reader.

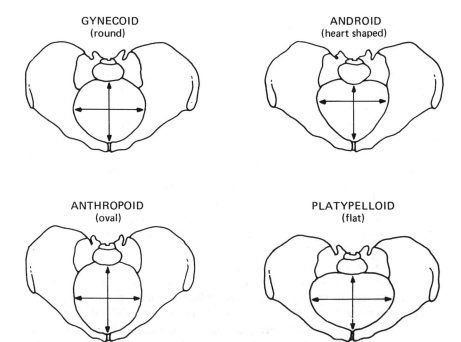

GYNECOID
(round)

ANDROID
(heart shaped)

ANTHROPOID
(oval)

PLATYPELLOID
(flat)

Figure 3-4. Pelvic types; shapes of pelvic inlets.

Review Questions

1. The normal female type pelvis is called _____ .

2. The three planes of the pelvis are: a. _____ ,
   b. _____ , and c. _____ .

3. Referring to the previous paragraph as necessary, the seven mechanisms of labor are: a. _____ ,
   b. _____ , c. _____ ,
   d. _____ , e. _____ ,
   f. _____ , and g. _____ .

Answers

1. The normal female type pelvis is called *gynecoid.*

2. The three planes of the pelvis are: a. *inlet,* b. *mid-pelvis,* and c.
   outlet.

3. The mechanisms of labor are: a. *descent,* b. *flexion,* c. *internal
   rotation,* d. *extension,* e. *restitution,* f. *external rotation,* and g.
   expulsion.

The Pelvic Inlet

The first mechanism for the fetal head is DESCENT into the inlet (pelvic brim) which is bordered by the symphysis pubis in front, the iliopectineal lines on the innominate bones on the sides, and the sacral promontory in the back (Fig. 3-5).

The diameter from front to back (anterior-posterior—AP) can be measured by the examiner. One or two digits (gloved) are inserted into the vagina and extended from below the symphysis pubis to the middle of the sacral promontory (a distinct projection on the upper portion of the sacrum). The distance from this prominence to the outside lower margin of the pubis is the *diagonal conjugate* (DC) and is *normally 12.5 cm*. In instances when the sacral promontory cannot be reached the examiner may indicate > 11 cm if he knows his fingers can reach 11 cm, or he may indicate NR for not reached.

The actual AP diameter that the fetus moves through is the inside measurement, the *obstetric conjugate* (OC), which is from the posterior superior aspect of the symphysis pubis to the sacral promontory. This diameter cannot be manually measured but is estimated by subtracting 1.5 cm from the DC. Therefore if the DC is 12.5 cm, the OC is 11.0 cm (12.5 − 1.5 = 11.0). The actual space available to the fetus in the AP diameter of the inlet (the OC) normally is 11.0 cm.

Without doing x-ray pelvimetry it is not possible to measure the transverse diameter of the inlet of the pelvis. But since a gynecoid pelvis has a round or slightly transverse oval inlet, and a circle (round) has consistently equal diameters, it can be assumed that if the AP diameter is 11.0 cm, the transverse diameter is also 11.0 cm; if the inlet is slightly oval, the transverse diameter is slightly longer.

The fetal head normally descends in the pelvic inlet in a transverse position (OT) or, less frequently, an oblique position—halfway between

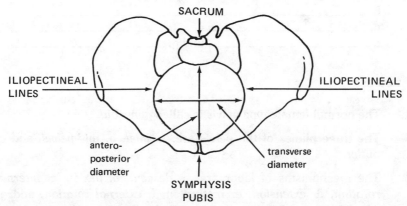

Figure 3-5. Inlet of gynecoid pelvis.

transverse and anterior or posterior. When the position of the head is OT the sagittal suture, which connects the anterior and posterior fontanels, is in the transverse diameter of the pelvis. The nonflexed head presents its occipitofrontal diameter, which is 11.0 cm. If the pelvic OC is also 11.0 cm, some molding will undoubtedly occur.

Review Questions

1. The boundaries of the pelvic inlet are: _____ , _____ , and _____ .

2. The (anteroposterior, transverse) diameter of the pelvic inlet is measurable manually. This diameter is called _____ _____ . Its length normally is _____ cm and is measured from _____ to _____ _____ .

3. The mechanism of labor that occurs in the inlet is _____ _____ .

4. The position of the head as it passes through the inlet is (anteroposterior, transverse). Circle one.

5. The diameter of the head that presents in the inlet is _____ _____ , which measures _____ cm.

6. What assumption can you make about the diameter of the head if it is to descend through the inlet of a gynecoid pelvis?

_____

_____

_____

Answers

1. The boundaries of the pelvic inlet are the *symphysis pubis,* the *iliopectineal lines,* and the *sacral promontory.*

2. The manually measurable *anteroposterior* diameter of the inlet is called the *diagonal conjugate* and measures *12.5* cm from the *subpubic arch* to the *middle of the sacral promontory.*

3. *Descent* occurs in the inlet.

4. The head enters the inlet in a *transverse* position.

5. The *occipitofrontal* diameter presents in the inlet and measures *11* cm.

6. The occipitofrontal diameter must be slightly smaller than the pelvic (usually transverse) diameter if the head is to move through this plane.

The Mid-Pelvis

In the mid-pelvis the head must bypass the lower margin of the symphysis pubis in front, the ischial spines on the sides, and the sacrum (S3-S4) in back (Fig. 3-6).

In order for there to be sufficient room for fetal descent there should be as few protrusions into the pelvis as possible. Therefore upon palpation the *sacrum* should be *curved* (outward—concave, hollow, deep) instead of flat, convex, or inwardly inclined. The *ischial spines* should be *nonprominent* or blunt, and the side walls parallel or nonconvergent.

Actual measurements of the mid-pelvis are not taken except by x-ray pelvimetry. A normal AP diameter is 11.5 cm, and a normal transverse diameter is 9.5 to 10.0 cm. Since the diameter of this plane in its lower portion is somewhat smaller than the inlet, the fetal neck experiences FLEXION, causing the smaller (9.5 cm) suboccipitobregmatic diameter to present.

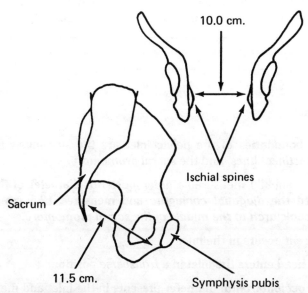

Figure 3-6. Mid-pelvis of gynecoid pelvis.

Review Questions

1. The three bones that border the mid-pelvic plane are: a. _____ _____ , b. _____ and c. _____ _____ .

2. By palpating, what ideal characteristics should be found about the:
   sacrum: _____
   ischial spines: _____
   side walls: _____

3. Circle the correct responses. The transverse diameter of the mid-pelvis is (smaller than, the same as, larger than) the transverse diameter of the inlet. Therefore the (occipitofrontal, suboccipito-bregmatic) diameter of the fetal head presents itself in this plane. In order for this to occur (descent, flexion, internal rotation) must take place.

Answers

1. The bones that border the mid-pelvis are: a. the *lower margin of the symphysis pubis;* b. the *ischial spines;* and c. the *sacrum.*

2. The sacrum should be curved; the spines, nonprominent; the side walls, nonconvergent.

3. The transverse diameter of the mid-pelvis is *smaller than* that of the inlet. Therefore the *suboccipitobregmatic* diameter presents as a result of *flexion.*

Remember to go back to the Pelvic Measurements Chart. Using the ideal normal findings, the *spines* are *nonprominent* and the *sacrum* is *curved.* Did you remember to fill in the normal pelvic type (gynecoid) and the normal DC (12.5 cm)?

The Pelvic Outlet

INTERNAL ROTATION of the head (from transverse to anterior position—OT to OA) occurs near or when the head reaches the pelvic outlet. This takes place simultaneously with descent and as a result of the need to be accommodated by the outlet diameters.

The outlet is the last pelvic plane the fetal head must pass through. It is bordered in front by the pubic arch, on the sides by the bi-ischial tuberosities, and in the back by the tip of the sacrum (coccyx). The transverse diameter is manually measurable between the *bi-ischial tuber-osities* (bitubs.); it usually measures about 11 cm. The anteroposterior diameter is determined by the *subpubic arch* (the angle under the symphysis pubis) and the coccyx. The diameter is adequate if a *90-degree angle* and a *movable coccyx* exist.

By the time the head passes through the outlet, it normally is flexed (a diameter of 9.5 cm) and rotated so the occiput (OA) lies beneath the symphysis pubis, and the sagittal suture (the suture line between the anterior and posterior fontanels) is in the anteroposterior diameter of the outlet. As the base of the occiput comes into direct contact with the inferior margin of the symphysis pubis, the occiput moves away from the sacrum. The resultant mechanism is EXTENSION and the head (caput) appears at and moves through the vaginal opening. The brow and face advance rapidly and appear in succession over the anterior margin of the perineum (posterior wall of vagina extending to rectum).

The head then falls back towards the anus. Once the head is out of the vagina the neck untwists, turning the head in the direction it previously was; this is known as RESTITUTION. Then the head is assisted to EXTERNALLY ROTATE completely to a transverse position as the shoulders rotate (anteroposterior) internally by essentially the same process that rotated the head internally. This orients the remainder of the body for the birth process. The anterior shoulder emerges under the pubic arch followed by the posterior shoulder. The remainder of the body, which is smaller in diameter, then delivers spontaneously (EXPULSION).

Review Questions

1. Descent and flexion have already occurred. What remaining mechanisms occur in or near the outlet? a. _____ , b. _____ , c. _____ , d. _____ , and e. _____ .

2. The pelvic measurements of concern in the outlet are associated with the following; give their ideal characteristics:
    bi-ischial tuberosities = _____cm.
    subpubic arch = _____degrees
    coccyx = _____ .

Answers

1. The mechanisms that occur in or near the outlet are: a. internal rotation, b. extension, c. restitution, d. external rotation, and e. expulsion.

2. Ideally the bi-ischial tuberosities are *11* cm, the subpubic arch is *90* degrees, and the coccyx is *movable.*

Now you are ready to fill in the remaining blanks of the Pelvic Measurements Chart. Your last answer (above) provides you with the correct information.

NURSING IMPLICATIONS
RELATED TO THE MECHANISMS OF LABOR

Using Predictive Data

The nurse has access to many data that are predictive of whether or not the normal mechanisms of labor are likely to occur or are occurring. The woman's obstetric history is one source of data. Consideration should be given to the size of her previous babies, the duration of those labors, and the occurrence of injury to the woman or babies during previous births. Since fetal weight and size usually have a direct relationship, a woman who has safely delivered an 8½-pound baby is not expected to have a difficult delivery this time, unless the estimated fetal weight (EFW) is larger. But the woman whose largest baby had a birth weight of 5 pounds, even though the labor was a short 5 hours, may have difficulty with an EFW of 7 pounds.

The pelvic measurements recorded on the chart are a source of information about possible pelvic contractures. If the DC is less than 12.5 cm, the fetus may continue to float above the pelvic inlet. If the spines are prominent or the sacrum flat or inwardly inclined, the fetus may have difficulty moving beyond the mid-pelvis (zero station). If the pubic arch is less than 90 degrees, the coccyx nonmovable, or the bitubs less than 11 cm, the outlet may be difficult for the normal size fetus to maneuver. Once the fetus passes a plane where difficulty had been expected, the characteristics of the next plane need to be considered.

Vaginal examinations provide further data about the fetal movement within the pelvis. In the presence of good uterine contractions there should be progressive cervical dilatation and fetal descent consistent with the norms established in the Friedman curves (see Chapter 4). Cervical effacement should be occurring without cervical edema because of pushing prior to complete dilatation. Molding of the fetal head is a normal finding, but the development of edema on the scalp (caput succedaneum) is not. The fetal position is also noted; ideally it moves from OT to OA.

Another source of data is the woman's expression of pain and tension. Both the nurse and the woman's designated support person should respond to these. Severe pain in the back is consistent with a fetal position of persistent occiput posterior (POP), which does not normally occur. (POP is common in android and anthropoid pelves.) Some back relief may be obtained by assuming a position other than supine—lateral, sitting, or knee-chest. Applying constant or intermittent sacral pressure may provide comfort. Heat (a moist towel) or cold (an ice bag) may also be beneficial when applied to the site of discomfort. A woman who is tense tightens her muscles, including those that line and support the pelvis. This causes resistance to fetal movement in a downward direction. Signs of emotional tension are uneven voice patterns, appearance of tears, inability to concentrate, or timid, fearful behavior. Relaxation techniques such as those used in Lamaze (see Chapter 8) should be used before medications are sought.

Review Questions

1. Why is it significant for the nurse to note the size and outcome of a woman's previous deliveries? _____
_____
_____

2. Which of the following are abnormal findings during a vaginal exam?
   a. cervical dilatation   d. fetal head molding
   b. cervical effacement   e. fetal head edema
   c. cervical edema   f. fetal position of POP

3. What measures can be taken to relieve back discomfort?
   a. _____
   b. _____
   c. _____

Answers

1. A woman who has delivered a baby of the same or smaller birth weight without adverse effects is expected to do the same this time.

2. During a vaginal exam it is abnormal to find: c. cervical edema, e. fetal head edema, and f. fetal position of POP.

3. To relieve back discomfort: a. change to positions other than supine; b. apply sacral pressure; and c. apply heat and/or cold to the site of discomfort.

Nursing Measures that Promote Descent

There are two physical principles that nurses can make use of when attempting to promote fetal descent: (1) gravity moves things downward; and (2) empty space will be filled.

When a pregnant woman is standing or sitting gravity encourages the fetus to descend. This position also brings the fetus forward so that the presenting fetal part is better aligned with the pelvic inlet and, therefore, able to move more easily into the pelvis.

Standing can be done in a number of ways: leaning against a wall, holding onto a side rail, or walking. One can stand or sit in a shower. Sitting can be done a. in bed with pillows and the head of the bed supporting the back, or leaning forward being supported by a padded bedside stand; b. in a comfortable chair, preferably a rocking chair; or c. on a bedpan or toilet. None of these positions should be assumed for a long period of time, because they become tiring.

The nurse can promote empty space by encouraging emptying of the bowel and bladder. When filled these organs take up considerable space in the pelvis. The bowel can be emptied with an enema if necessary. (This might also stimulate the labor; see Chapter 5.) The bladder should be emptied spontaneously if possible every 2 to 3 hours, or via catheterization, if the bladder is palpable and the woman is unable to empty it on her own.

Review Questions

1. If a woman is tired of being on her feet, identify two alternate positions a nurse could suggest that might promote fetal descent.
    a. _____
    b. _____

2. How does having a woman in labor void every 2 to 3 hours promote fetal descent? _____
    _____

Answers

1. In addition to standing, a nurse could suggest sitting a. in a shower, b. in a bed leaning backward supported with pillows; or c. in bed leaning forward, d. in a chair, or e. on a bedpan or toilet, to promote fetal descent.
2. Frequent voiding provides space that is otherwise occupied by a filling bladder.

Nursing Measures that Provide Changes in Fetal Position

For many years nurses have recognized the benefits of altering a woman's position during labor. For one, she is more comfortable. For another, position changes often spontaneously rotate the fetus to a more desirable position.

There are theoretical reasons why a fetus will rotate when the mother assumes certain postures. The back is the heaviest, densest part of the fetal body except for the head. Given time, the back will rotate to the lower side of the maternal abdomen placing the lighter more buoyant small parts of the fetus on the upper side. A woman who lies on her back is likely to cause the fetus to assume a posterior (OP) position. By assuming a Sims' position she facilitates fetal rotation to OA. (Sims' position is semiprone on one side [e.g., left] with that [left] arm behind the back, and the chest inclined forward, the legs flexed with the upper [right] knee closest to the chest.) This position also promotes less pain associated with uterine contractions and greater efficiency from the contractions.

Claire Andrews, in her 1980 article in the Journal of Nurse-Midwifery, recommends additional nursing measures to rotate a fetus to OA. Get the mother in a hands-and-knees posture with hands fisted to prevent wrist fatigue. Pelvic rock 10 times slowly and rhythmically. Then with lower back arched towards the ceiling, mother or coach gently but deeply stroke 10 times from back to front on the side of the fetal back (which is the same as the occiput), continuing as far as possible to the other side.

> If ROP or ROT, stroke from right to left.
> If OP, stroke right to left.
> If LOP or LOT, stroke from left to right.

This combination of pelvic rocking and stroking is continued for 10 minutes at a time. Rest periods are taken with the mother lying in Sims' position and then the above exercises are repeated. For the fetus who is ROT, the mother rests in Sims' position on her left side to encourage the fetus to rotate (90 degrees forward to OA). For the fetus who is ROP she rests in Sims' position on her right side to encourage the fetus to rotate (less than 180 degrees to OA).

If rotation is necessary it should be attempted early in labor to promote comfort. In some instances, for example, if the inlet has a contracted anterior segment, rotation from OP should not be attempted until the head has passed the inlet. In other pelves, a position other than OA may be advantageous for fetal movement through the pelvis; for example, OP in anthropoid and OT in platypelloid. Until individual nurses are well versed in pelvic particulars, they will need to accept the guidance they receive from attending physicians.

Review Question

Explain 3 ways to promote changes in fetal position:

a. _____

_____

b. _____

_____

c. _____

_____

Answer

To promote changes in fetal position, do the following:

a. Have the mother lie on the side to which the heavy back (occiput) ideally would turn; for example, for OA have her be as near prone as possible (via Sims' or knee-chest position).
b. Have her pelvic rock while on hands and knees.
c. Have mother (or someone else) stroke the fetal back in the direction in which the fetus should turn.

CONCLUSION

If you are like most readers, you would benefit from seeing a fetus go through the mechanisms of labor. If you have access to models of a fetal head and pelvis, go through the motions that have been described in this chapter. The real test of your understanding of the mechanisms of labor will come in your application of this knowledge—whether it be during the care of a woman in labor, or your explanation of the mechanisms to another person.

BIBLIOGRAPHY

ANDREWS, CM: *Changing fetal position.* J Nurs-Midw 25(1):7, 1980.

ANDREWS, CM: *Nursing interventions to change a malpositioned fetus.* Advances in Nursing Science 3(2):53, 1981.

BENSON, RC: *Current Obstetric and Gynecologic Diagnosis and Treatment,* ed 3. Lange Medical Publications, Los Altos, Calif, 1980.

CARR, KC: *Obstetric practices which protect against neonatal morbidity: Focus on maternal position in labor and birth.* Birth and the Family Journal 7(4):249, 1980.

McKay, SR: *Maternal position during labor and birth.* J Obstet Gynecol Neonatal Nurs 9:288, 1980.

Meissner, JE: *Predicting a patient's anxiety level during labor: A two-part assessment tool.* Nurs 80 10:50, 1980.

Oxorn, H: *Oxorn-Foote: Human Labor and Birth,* ed 4. Appleton-Century-Crofts, New York, 1980.

Roberts, J: *Alternative positions for childbirth—Part I: First stage of labor.* J Nurs-Midw 25(4):11, 1980.

POST-TEST

1. The following landmarks are significant in the various planes of the pelvis. Identify the plane in which each landmark is located and which diameter (anteroposterior or transverse) it influences.

	PLANE	DIAMETER
Bi-ischial tuberosities		
Posterior superior margin of symphysis pubis		
Coccyx		
Ischial spines		
Subpubic arch		

2. Describe the ideal passage of the fetus through the pelvis. Include the mechanisms and diameters of pelvis (when appropriate).

_____

_____

_____

_____

_____

_____

_____

_____

_____

3. Put a check mark (✓) in front of those items that indicate ideal characteristics of the pelvis:

_____ DC of 10.5 cm   _____ convergent side walls

_____ hollow sacrum   _____ bituberosities of 7.5

_____ blunt (ischial) spines   cm

_____ movable coccyx   _____ arch of 80 degrees

                                             _____ android type

4. Mrs. Beebe appears comfortable, although vaginal examination indicates she is 5 cm, 0 station, ROP. Her previous labor had an

uncomplicated delivery of a 4-pound baby; the current EFW is 6 pounds. Her pelvic measurements are: DC 11 cm; spines nonprominent; sacrum hollow; arch 85 degrees; bitubs 11 cm; coccyx movable; Type gynecoid.

a. Give at least 3 reasons why you anticipate she will undergo the normal mechanisms of labor despite a few problematic data:

(1) _____

(2) _____

(3) _____

b. Indicate 2 ways you might encourage fetal descent:

(1) _____

(2) _____

c. What 3 measures might a nurse take to promote ideal fetal position?

(1) _____

(2) _____

(3) _____

Answers

1. Bi-ischial tuberosities: outlet, transverse
    Posterior superior margin of symphysis pubis: inlet, anteroposterior
    Coccyx: outlet, anteroposterior
    Ischial spines: mid-pelvis, transverse
    Subpubic arch: outlet, anteroposterior.

2. The occipitofrontal diameter of the head descends into the transverse diameter (occasionally oblique) of the inlet of the gynecoid pelvis. It descends further into the mid-plane, flexing to the smaller suboccipitobregmatic diameter. The head usually internally rotates from transverse to anteroposterior diameter when it reaches the outlet. The occiput moves under the symphysis pubis and extends, bringing the head out through the vaginal opening. Then restitution of the head occurs and the head externally rotates to a transverse position, orienting the remainder of the body for expulsion.

3. Ideal characteristics of the pelvis are hollow sacrum, blunt spines, movable coccyx.

4. a. Although the baby is approximately 2 pounds larger than her previous one, the baby has (1) already moved through the inlet (past the small DC) and is in the (2) mid-pelvis (zero station), which appears adequate (considering the spines and sacrum). The other slightly small area is the 85-degree arch; (3) a relatively small baby (6 pounds) should be accommodated by this

(4) pelvic outlet, since all the other measurements (bitubs and coccyx) are ideal. The OP fetal position is not ideal but is (5) not creating any apparent discomfort. (The Friedman curve should be assessed for abnormal cervical dilatation and descent patterns.)

b. Fetal descent could be encouraged by (1) allowing the force of gravity to work (have the mother stand or sit), and (2) providing more pelvic space by keeping the bowel and bladder empty.

c. The fetus should be rotated from ROP to OA. The nurse should encourage the mother to (1) lie frequently on her right side in a Sims' position. Periodically, the mother can (2) get up on her hands and knees and pelvic rock. She can also (3) stroke her abdomen (fetus) from right to left encouraging rotation.

CHAPTER **4**

USING LABOR GRAPHS
TO GUIDE
NURSING CARE

Janet S. Malinowski

Graphing the course of a labor is an efficient way to document cervical dilatation and fetal descent patterns. By knowing what is normal and what is abnormal on the graph, the nurse can help to provide a safer outcome for the mother and her baby. This chapter presents the basic information that the nurse should know about labor graphs.

OBJECTIVES

Upon completion of this chapter, the reader will be able to:

1. Identify the phases of the S curve seen in a normal cervical dilatation curve.
2. Use a reference that designates the normal time limits for the two dilatation phases.
3. Diagram and state the criteria for, causes of, and interventions for the following abnormal dilatation patterns: precipitous labor, prolonged latent phase, slow slope active phase, and arrest of the active phase.
4. Differentiate between normal and abnormal descent patterns in a nullipara and a multipara.
5. State the criteria for protracted descent and arrest of descent.
6. Recognize the nursing interventions pertinent to prolonged labor.
7. Given specific data about a patient in labor, interpret the labor curves and explain the theory that supports the interpretation.
8. Correctly plot all given data on a graph and draw conclusions about the meaning of the data and the appropriate nursing interventions to be taken.

Methodology of Graphing Labor Patterns

In 1964 Emanuel A. Friedman introduced his analysis of the labor patterns of 500 nulliparous (first labor) and 500 multiparous (other than first labor) women. He graphically recorded labor patterns and established normal time limits for the various phases of labor. Since then tens of thousands of labors have been analyzed. By recognizing an abnormal pattern, the nurse can prevent a dangerous situation by using appropriate interventions.

Using Friedman's method the labor pattern is plotted on square ruled paper, with each square being of equal value. The left vertical scale indicates the ascending cervical dilatation (in centimeters from 0 to 10) and is marked with a small circle. The right scale, the descending station (going from minus to plus), is marked with an X. The horizontal axis indicates the time in hours—from onset of labor until complete dilatation. Each time a vaginal exam is performed, the cervical dilatation and station for that time are graphed. It is also helpful to record any other significant interventions (for example, rupture of membranes, administration of medication) at the time they are performed.

The time of onset of labor is not clear-cut. A common misconception is that rupture of membranes or occasional contractions indicate the onset. Most authorities say that the onset of labor is the time when the woman experiences *regular* uterine contractions that lead to progressive cervical changes. Until a regular pattern occurs, true labor has not begun.

Review Questions

1. The results of each vaginal exam are spaced on vertical lines according to the: _____ .

2. The onset of labor should be plotted as the time of: _____
   _____ .

Answers

1. The results of vaginal exams are recorded according to the time at which the exams are performed, with each vertical line being worth an equal amount of time.
2. The onset of labor should be plotted as the time of the beginning of regular contractions, *not* rupture of membranes or occasional contractions.

Phases of the S Curve
in a Normal Cervical Dilatation Pattern

Friedman found that the normal labor pattern of cervical dilatation has an S-shaped curve and that this curve could be divided into two phases: latent and active (Fig. 4-1).

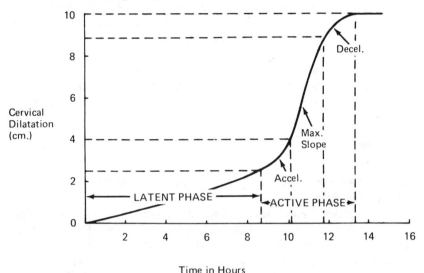

Time in Hours

Figure 4-1. Mean labor curve of a nullipara.

The *latent phase* extends from the onset of regular uterine contractions to the beginning of the active phase—around 3 cm dilatation. The nullipara may normally spend up to 20 hours in this phase, the multipara 14 hours; although as Table 4-1 indicates, the mean time is considerably less. During this phase the nurse needs to help the laboring woman to relax, both physically and mentally. This is the time to establish rapport, to familiarize the woman with her surroundings, and to discuss the expected occurrences of labor.

The latent phase is graphically flat. The cervix becomes more effaced but only dilates slightly. The duration of the phase is sensitive to extra-

TABLE 4-1 Means of Time in Stage I

	Nullipara	Multipara
Latent phase	6.4 hrs. (20.1)*	4.8 hrs. (13.6)*
Active phase	4.6 hrs. (11.7)*	2.4 hrs. (5.2) *

*Maximum limit of normal
Adapted from FRIEDMAN, E: *Labor: Clinical Evaluation and Management*, ed 2. Appleton-Century-Crofts, New York, 1978, p 49.

neous factors; a sedative would prolong it, whereas an enema (stimulant) might shorten it. Although normally more than half the time spent in labor involves the latent phase, its length is no indication of how long the active phase will be.

During the *active phase* the graphic curve begins to incline steeply; the phase ends at complete cervical dilatation (10 cm—the end of Stage I). The nurse should anticipate that numerous signs of progress (refer to Chapter 1) will occur during this phase. Increased pain will require comfort measures, relaxation techniques, and possibly analgesia. Up to 12 hours might be normally spent in this phase by the nullipara; up to 6 hours, for the multiparous woman. See Table 4-1 for the mean times.

The active phase is subdivided into three parts. During the *acceleration phase* the cervix begins to dilate more rapidly. During the *phase of maximum slope* the inclination (slope) is steep; the major portion of cervical dilatation occurs here. Last is the *deceleration phase*—a slowing down in the rate of cervical dilatation just prior to complete dilatation. Often this phase is very short or absent. Unless the cervical dilatation is assessed at exactly the right time, a slowing down in the dilatation rate may not be evident.

The S-shaped curve seen in Figure 4-1 is normal for both nulliparous and multiparous women. But the length of time that each one spends in each phase differs; refer to Table 4-1. The mean length of Stage I for the nulliparous woman is 11 hours, whereas the mean for the multiparous woman is approximately 7 hours. The graph does not enable the nurse to predict the exact time of delivery, but it does document progress, or the lack of progress, in labor.

Review Question

Stage I is divided into phases in the following way:
(1) _____
(2) _____
    a. _____
    b. _____
    c. _____

Answer

Stage I is divided into (1) the latent phase and (2) the active phase, which is subdivided into a. acceleration phase, b. phase of maximum slope, and c. deceleration phase.

Abnormal Cervical Dilatation Patterns

Friedman identified several abnormal cervical dilatation patterns. *Precipitous labor* involves an extremely short Stage I. On the other hand, the *prolonged latent phase, slow slope* (or *protracted*) *active phase, and arrest of the active phase* all involve time beyond the established normal limits for a specific phase. See Figure 4-2 for a graphic view of these abnormal patterns.

DEFINITIONS, CAUSES, AND INTERVENTIONS FOR ABNORMAL DILATATION PATTERNS

Precipitous Labor

Labor in which complete dilatation occurs in less than 2 or 3 hours is generally called *precipitous labor*. Friedman is more specific and defines it as rates of dilatation greater than 5 cm per hour in nulliparas, and 10 cm per hour in multiparas. Less resistance from the maternal soft tissues makes precipitous labor more likely in the multipara than in the nullipara. Very rapid cervical dilatation is usually accompanied by very rapid fetal descent. Following repeated vaginal examinations both of these occurrences should be detectable graphically.

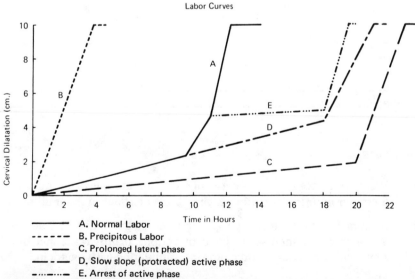

Figure 4-2. Labor curves of nulliparous women.

Nurses should suspect this pattern when uterine contractions are very frequent and intense. Careful assessment should be made of the fetal heart rate, since there is a significant decrease in oxygen supply when the mother has vigorous contractions. Uterine rupture could result. (Signs to look for are severe, abrupt abdominal pain, cessation of contractions, vaginal bleeding, shock, and decreasing or nonexistent fetal heart rate.) Uterine stimulation with oxytocin is often a causative factor. (See Chapter 5.) If oxytocin is being used, it must immediately be discontinued. Other interventions rarely slow this labor pattern. The nurse should prepare for a supervised, controlled, and preferably sterile delivery and at the same time meet the psychologic needs of a woman undergoing a very stressful labor.

Review Questions

1. Precipitous labor involves cervical dilatation at rates of greater than _____ cm per hour in the nullipara and _____ cm per hour in the multipara.

2. Factors that cause this very rapid cervical dilatation and fetal descent are:
   a. _____
   b. _____
   c. _____

3. List five nursing interventions that should occur during a precipitous labor.
   a. _____
   b. _____
   c. _____
   d. _____
   e. _____

Answers

1. Precipitous labor involves cervical dilatation at rates of greater than 5 cm per hour in the nullipara and 10 cm per hour in the multipara.

2. Factors that cause this very rapid cervical dilatation and fetal descent are: a. frequent, intense uterine contractions; b. little resistance from maternal soft tissues; and c. uterine stimulation with oxytocin.

3. Nursing interventions during a precipitous labor include:
   a.   assess fetal heart rate for signs of distress;

b.   observe for signs of uterine rupture;

c.   stop oxytocin infusion immediately (if oxytocin is being used);

d.   facilitate a supervised, controlled, sterile delivery;

e.   provide psychologic support.

Prolonged Latent Phase

According to Friedman, a *prolonged latent phase* is 20 hours or more in a nullipara and 14 hours or more in a multipara. The ambiguous definition of onset of labor makes diagnosis of this abnormality especially difficult.

The most frequent causes of prolonged latent phase are excessive sedation (via narcotic analgesic or sedative); anesthesia; unripe (thick, uneffaced) cervix; and false labor. Another cause, less frequent, is malposition, specifically occiput posterior (OP) and occiput transverse (OT).

Ironically an effective terminator of this prolonged phase is an initial dose of morphine sulfate, 15 mg subcutaneously followed 20 minutes later by an additional 10 mg of morphine if needed. The intent is to temporarily stop contractions and provide therapeutic rest. Frequently, several treatments are tried; for example, ambulation; enema; artificial rupture of membranes (of questionable effectiveness); and, if still necessary, administration of oxytocin, which may be effective in stimulating uterine contractions and cervical dilatation. (See Chapter 5.) Cesarean delivery, however, is not a treatment for this abnormality.

A prolonged latent phase supposedly does not endanger the woman in labor and her fetus. But if it goes untreated, it often causes maternal exhaustion and low morale, and possibly dehydration and intrauterine infection (if membranes are ruptured).

Review Questions

1.   A prolonged latent phase is one that is greater than _____ hours in a nullipara and greater than _____ hours in a multipara.

2.   Prolonged latent phase is closely associated with:

    a. _____ , b. _____ ,

    c. _____ .

3.   Two general medical approaches to prolonged latent phase are:

    a. _____ and b. _____ .

4.   Possible complications of prolonged latent phase are

    a. _____ , b. _____ ,

    c. _____ , and d. _____ .

Answers

1. A prolonged latent phase is greater than 20 hours in a nullipara and greater than 14 hours in a multipara.
2. Prolonged latent phase is closely associated with excessive sedation, anesthesia, unripe cervix, and false labor.
3. Two general medical approaches to prolonged latent phase are
    a. stop contractions and provide rest (for example, with morphine),
    b. stimulate labor with one or more methods.
4. Possible complications of prolonged latent phase are maternal exhaustion, low morale/discouragement, dehydration, and intra-uterine infection.

Slow Slope Active Phase

Another abnormal labor pattern is the *slow slope* (or *protracted*) *active phase*. (Refer to Figure 4-2 for a graphic representation.) It is also called primary dysfunctional labor. By definition it has a maximum slope of dilatation of 1.2 cm or less per hour in the nullipara and 1.5 cm or less per hour in the multipara.

Frequently a fetal position of OP or OT exists and is thought to contribute to the poor uterine forces. This malposition, as well as fetopelvic disproportion and too early amniotomy, appear to be the primary causes of this abnormal dilatation pattern. It occurs more frequently during a first labor owing to soft tissue resistance in the pelvis; usually it does not recur in succeeding labors.

Despite contractions that become stronger and longer, the slowly progressing cervical dilatation curve is difficult to alter, even with uterine stimulation or amniotomy. In many women, the dilatation eventually stops, and a cesarean delivery is required. In others a constant, abnormally slow dilatation continues.

The woman finds this prolonged labor to be even more uncomfortable than she had anticipated. But as long as she makes some progress and there is no fetal distress, only supportive care should be given. The danger to the fetus occurs mainly at the time of vaginal delivery when midforceps may cause trauma.

Review Questions

1. The slow slope active phase is also called the _____ active phase.

2. The slow slope active phase exists when dilatation is _____ or less in the nullipara and _____ cm or less per hour in the multipara.

3. What are the primary causes of a slow slope active phase?
   a. _____ c. _____
   b. _____ d. _____

4. Why would you expect the patient to become frustrated? _____

Answers

1. The slow slope active phase is also called the protracted active phase.

2. The slow slope active phase exists when dilatation is 1.2 cm or less per hour in the nullipara and 1.5 cm or less per hour in a multipara.

3. The primary causes of a slow slope active phase are malposition, fetopelvic disproportion, too early amniotomy, and soft tissue resistance (in the nullipara).

4. The patient becomes frustrated because the contractions become stronger and longer, but there is little progress and no interventions help to speed up the labor.

Arrest of the Active Phase

In (secondary) *arrest of the active phase,* previously advancing cervical dilatation stops for 2 hours or more. A variation of this abnormality is a prolonged deceleration phase (that is, greater than 3 hours in nulliparas; greater than 1 hour in multiparas).

Fetopelvic disproportion is the major cause of this abnormality. Excessive sedation, fetal malposition, and anesthesia are also common causes.

For those women under the influence of medication, providing time for rest while the effects of medication wear off usually results in labor progress. If the fetopelvic relationship is favorable, oxytocin stimulation may also be used. For those with bony dystocia (inadequate fetopelvic relationship) a cesarean delivery is necessary.

Review Questions

1. Arrest of the active phase is defined as _____
   _____ .

2. Four possible causes of arrest of the active phase are:
   a. _____ c. _____
   b. _____ d. _____

3. What are three possible methods of treatment for arrest of the active phase? a. _____ , b. _____ , and c. _____ .

Answers

1. Arrest of the active phase of dilatation is no progress in dilatation for 2 hours or more during the active phase.

2. Possible causes of arrest in the active phase are fetopelvic disproportion, excessive sedation, fetal malposition, and anesthesia.

3. Possible methods of treatment are rest and support, uterine stimulation, and cesarean delivery.

DESCENT PATTERNS

Thus far we have focused only on the graphic pattern of cervical dilatation. Descent of the fetus should also be graphed and analyzed for normal and abnormal patterns.

The normal descent pattern will be considered first. Descent is the first requisite for the birth of the fetus. When the fetal head has descended so that its greatest biparietal diameter is at, or has passed, the pelvic inlet, the head is *engaged*. (At this point the occiput is near the spines, almost at zero station. Refer to Chapter 3 for additional information.) In the nullipara, engagement usually occurs at or before the onset of labor. In the multipara, once engagement occurs further descent occurs rapidly; engagement may not take place until the active phase of dilatation. Descent is brought about by four forces: (1) pressure of the amniotic fluid; (2) direct pressure of the fundus upon the buttocks; (3) contraction of the abdominal muscles; and (4) extension and straightening of the body of the fetus.

Review Questions

1. What is the difference between the occurrence of engagement in the nullipara as compared with engagement in the multipara? _____
_____

2. Identify the four forces that cause descent:
   a. _____ c. _____
   b. _____ d. _____

Answers

1. In the nullipara engagement occurs at or before the onset of labor. In the multipara engagement may not take place until the active phase of dilatation has begun; thereafter descent occurs rapidly.

2. The forces that bring about descent are pressure of the amniotic fluid, direct pressure of the fundus upon the buttocks, contraction of the abdominal muscles, and extension and straightening of the body of the fetus.

Now look at the normal descent patterns illustrated in Figure 4-3 for the nullipara and in Figure 4-4 for the multipara. Both show the normal S-shaped curve of the cervical dilatation pattern. They also show the descent curve. On the right side the station is calibrated as −1, 0, +1, and so forth; the distance between each point (for example, −1 to 0) is 1 cm. At the top of the graph the descent curve is divided into a latent, an accelerated, and a maximum slope phase. This is not exactly the same as the dilatation curve (at the bottom). The shaded area shows that *the maximum slope in dilatation and the onset of acceleration in descent occur at the same time.* The average rates at the right of the graphs, determined by Friedman, are intended primarily as a reference. The rate of descent (like the rate of dilatation) is normally faster in the multipara than in the nullipara. And, the rate of descent is considerably

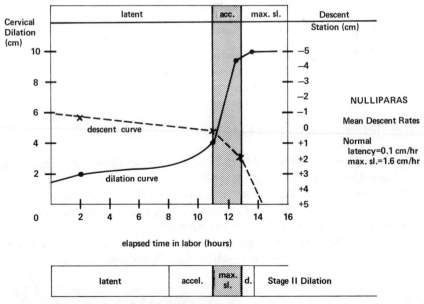

Figure 4-3. Normal pattern in nullipara.

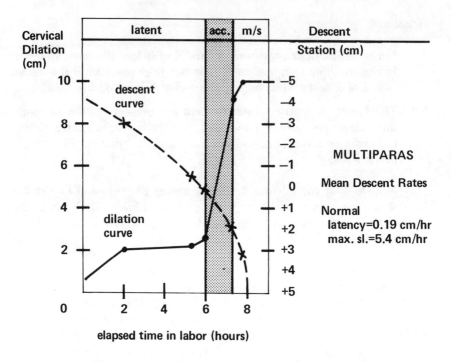

Figure 4-4. Normal pattern in multipara.

faster during the maximum slope than in the latent phase. Note the differences in the two descent curves—the initial station, the occurrence of engagement (−1 to 0 station), and the rate of descent.

Two Abnormal Descent Patterns

Abnormalities in the descent pattern occur twice as often in the nullipara. Two abnormal rates are worth learning:

A *protracted descent pattern* exists when the rate of descent in the active phase* of descent is less than 1.0 cm per hour in the nullipara, and less than 2.0 cm per hour in the multipara.

An *arrest of descent* during the active phase of descent—no linear advancement of station—exists when there is no progress for 1 hour or more.

---

*The active phase is composed of both the accelerated and maximum slope phases.

There are two major causes of abnormal descent patterns: fetopelvic disproportion and malposition (OP and OT being the most common). Both causes make it difficult, if not impossible, for the fetus to fit through the pelvis. Excessive sedation or anesthesia is another possible cause, since sedation or anesthesia reduces uterine fundal pressure and abdominal muscular pressure.

Minor fetopelvic disproportion may be spontaneously resolved by molding (overriding of the bones) of the fetal head. Rotation of the malpositioned head to OA may be encouraged by proper positioning of the mother (see Chapter 3), or manual rotation by hand or forceps. Given time, the effects of a sedative or anesthesia will decrease and normal descent forces will begin to work again. The nurse can be instrumental in facilitating these interventions and explaining their purpose. If descent beyond zero station does not occur, cesarean delivery will be necessary.

Review Questions

1. In a normal labor pattern, the onset of the acceleration of descent occurs at the same time as _____ .

2. In a nullipara the descent rate is (faster than, same as, slower than) that in a multipara. (Choose one.)

3. Abnormalities in descent patterns occur (more often, less often) in nulliparas than in multiparas. (Choose one.)

4. Complete the following statements for both the nullipara and multipara:
   a. A protracted descent pattern exists when the rate of descent in the active phase of descent is _____ in a nullipara and _____ in a multipara.
   b. An arrest of descent during the active phase of descent exists when _____ .

5. Considering the major causes of abnormal descent patterns, list three ways a nurse can facilitate descent:
   a. _____
   b. _____
   c. _____

Answers

1. The onset of the acceleration of descent occurs at the same time as the maximum slope in cervical dilatation.

2. A nullipara has a slower descent rate than a multipara.

3.   Abnormalities in descent patterns occur more often in the nullipara.

4.   a.   A protracted descent pattern in a nullipara is less than 1.0 cm per hour; in a multipara a protracted descent pattern is less than 2 cm per hour.
     b.   An arrest of descent is no progress for one hour or more.

5.   Ways a nurse can facilitate descent include:
     a.   allow time for molding of the fetal head to occur or for the inhibiting effects of sedatives/anesthesia to wear off
     b.   position the mother to facilitate fetal rotation to OA
     c.   explain rationale for interventions and give supportive care.

NURSING INTERVENTIONS IN THE PRESENCE OF PROLONGED LABOR

No matter what the cause of prolongation may be, the nurse as caretaker is primary assessor and legally responsible for recording her findings and interventions. Periodically assessing the uterine contractions and other signs of progress, she compares these findings with those on the labor graph. Astute noninvasive observations by the nurse can often minimize the number of vaginal exams and thereby decrease the risk of intrauterine infection, especially following rupture of membranes. Any inconsistencies, for example, strong frequent uterine contractions but no progress in cervical dilatation, need to be shared with the doctor. Nursing measures that might promote cervical dilatation and fetal descent and rotation, such as ambulation and periodic position changes, are discussed in Chapters 3, 5, and 9.

Other nursing measures during prolonged labor involve fetal response, fluid intake and output, medications, and psychologic needs. The nurse periodically evaluates the fetal response, noting signs of fetal distress that warrant immediate intervention. (Refer to Chapter 2 for uterine contraction and fetal heart rate assessment.) In order to prevent dehydration (evident by acetonuria), which could occur from prolonged labor, she provides at least 2500 ml of fluid daily. Usually an IV glucose solution is preferred, since there is poor digestion of food during labor, and vomiting with subsequent aspiration is possible. Adequate emptying of the bladder and bowel facilitates fetal descent and decreases discomfort. Judicious administration of sedation and analgesia is necessary, since excessive medication may interfere with contractions and harm the fetus. The nurse must tend to the woman's psychologic needs—bolstering morale, offering warranted encouragement, and avoiding remarks that might worry the woman, since anxiety may slow the labor process.

Review Question

Reread the previous two paragraphs. By underlining or highlighting in some other way, indicate the nine nursing interventions identified.

Answers

Nursing interventions that should be taken during prolonged labor include:
1. record all findings and interventions;
2. assess uterine contractions and other indications of progress;
3. compare findings with those recorded on labor graph;
4. share inconsistencies (abnormal findings) with doctor;
5. evaluate fetal response;
6. prevent dehydration;
7. empty bladder and bowel;
8. judiciously administer sedatives and analgesia;
9. tend to psychologic needs decreasing anxiety.

CONCLUSION

With basic knowledge of normal and abnormal patterns of dilatation and descent, you should be able to function more efficiently in a labor area. If labor graphs are not used in the area where you work, you should at least be able to draw a mental picture of what is occurring. Based on this image, you can determine whether the pattern is normal or abnormal, and if intervention is necessary.

BIBLIOGRAPHY

FRIEDMAN, EA: *Labor: Clinical Evaluation and Management,* ed 2. Appleton-Century-Crofts, New York, 1978.

OLDS, SB, ET AL: *Obstetric Nursing.* Addison-Wesley, Menlo Park, Calif, 1980, pp 485–493.

OXORN, H: *Human Labor and Birth,* ed 4. Appleton-Century-Crofts, New York, 1980.

SEHGAL, NN: *Early detection of abnormal labor using the Friedman labor graph.* Postgrad Med 68(13):189, 1980.

POST-TEST

1. Put a check mark (✓) in front of those statements that indicate an abnormal pattern. Following those checked statements, briefly explain why the pattern is abnormal.

_____ a.   A nullipara whose labor is 13 hours in length.

_____

_____

_____ b.   A nullipara whose latent phase is 21 hours.

_____

_____

_____ c.   A nullipara who is at zero station two weeks before the onset of labor.

_____

_____

_____ d.   A labor that is three hours in length.

_____

_____

_____ e.   A multipara who is in the active phase for eight hours.

_____

_____

_____ f.   A nullipara who remains at 6 cm for five hours.

_____

_____

_____ g.   A descent pattern that begins active deceleration as the cervix dilates the most rapidly.

_____

_____

_____ h.   A dilatation pattern that does not show a deceleration phase.

_____

_____

2. Fill in the blanks, identifying the various phases in this labor graph.

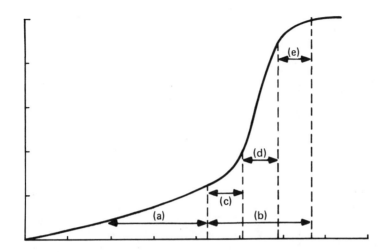

a. _____

b. _____

c. _____

d. _____

e. _____

3. **Diagram on the graphs provided and describe in words the following patterns. Place your drawings on top of the normal curves already drawn.**

Diagram: **Word Description:**
a. Prolonged latent phase:

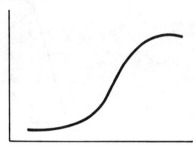

b. Protracted active phase:

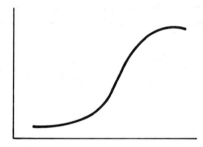

c. Arrest of the active phase:

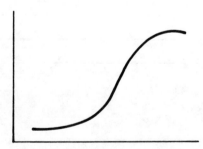

4. **Describe the following as they apply to both the nullipara and multipara.**
   a. Protracted descent pattern: _____
   _____
   _____

   b. Arrest of descent: _____
   _____
   _____

5. Below you will find the data from two labor records. Time, cervical dilatation, and station are provided. Put these data on graphs. Analyze the graphs for their patterns. Then summarize your interpretations in writing. Include nursing interventions if they are other than routine care.

Patient A: a multipara.

Time	Cervical Dilatation	Station
12:00 Mn	2	−2
5:30 A.M.	2	−1
6:00 A.M.	2–3	0
7:00 A.M.	7	+1
7:30 A.M.	9	+2
7:45 A.M.	complete	+4, caput showing

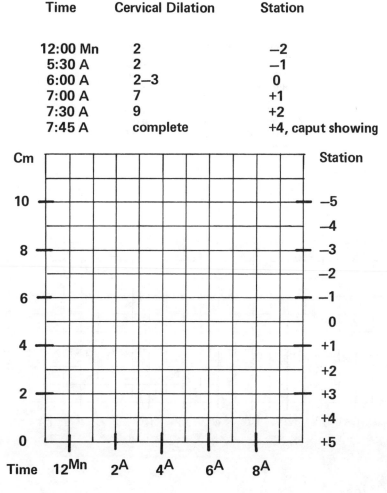

Time	Cervical Dilation	Station
12:00 Mn	2	−2
5:30 A	2	−1
6:00 A	2–3	0
7:00 A	7	+1
7:30 A	9	+2
7:45 A	complete	+4, caput showing

Interpretation: _____

_____

_____

_____

_____

Patient B: a nullipara.

Time	Cervical Dilatation	Station
12:00 Mn	1–2	−1 to 0
4:00 A.M.	2	0
8:00 A.M.	2–3	0 to +1
11:00 A.M.	4	0 to +1
12:00 N	5	0 to +1
2:00 P.M.	6	0 to +1
3:00 P.M.	7	+1
4:00 P.M.	7	+1
4:30 P.M.	8	+2
5:00 P.M.	10	+2

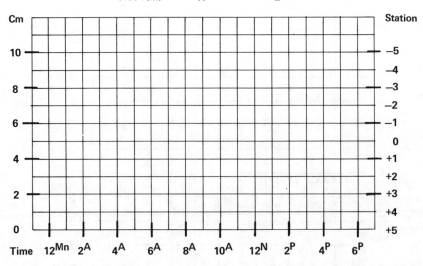

Time	Cervical Dilation	Station
12:00 Mn	1–2	−1 to 0
4:00 A.M.	2	0
8:00 A.M.	2–3	0 to +1
11:00 A.M.	4	0 to +1
12:00 N	5	0 to +1
2:00 P.M.	6	0 to +1
3:00 P.M.	7	+1
4:00 P.M.	7	+1
4:30 P.M.	8	+2
5:00 P.M.	10	+2

Interpretation: _____

_____
_____
_____
_____

Answers to Post-Test

1. The following statements should be checked:
    b. 21 hours is prolonged.
    d. This is a precipitous labor and therefore abnormal.
    e. Cervical dilatation in the active phase is from 4 to 10 cm (or is equal to 6 cm). Less than 1.5 cm per hour in the active phase for a multipara is a slow slope. Six divided by 1.5 = 4 hours; greater than 4 hours in the active phase is a slow slope active phase.
    f. Remaining at 6 cm for 2 hours or more indicates an arrest.
2. a. latent phase; b. active phase; c. accelerated phase; d. phase of maximum slope; e. deceleration phase.
3. For the drawings refer back to Figure 4-2. The prolonged latent phase is generally flat with 20 or more hours for the nullipara and 14 or more hours for the multipara. The protracted active phase involves slow movement through the active phase with 1.2 cm or less per hour cervical dilatation for the nullipara and 1.5 cm or less per hour cervical dilatation for the multipara. Arrest of the active phase of labor is indicated by no progress for at least 2 hours.
4. a. A protracted descent pattern exists when the rate in the active phase of descent is less than 1.0 cm per hour in the nullipara and less than 2 cm per hour in the multipara.
    b. An arrest of descent during the active phase of descent exists when there is no progress for 1 hour or more.

5. Patient A:

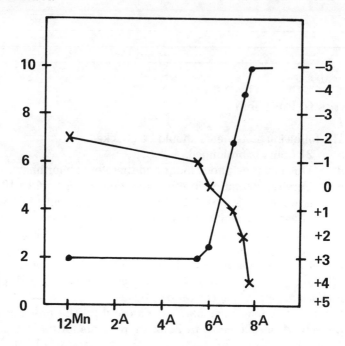

Patient B:

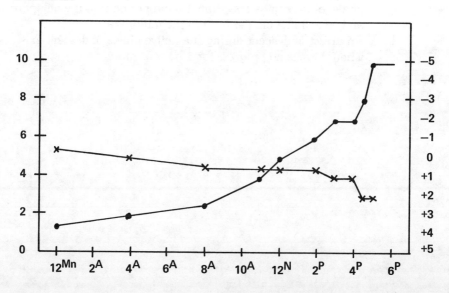

NURSING CARE OF THE LABOR PATIENT

Patient A: This is a normal labor pattern for a multipara. Stage I is almost 8 hours long; a normal length is approximately 6½ to 8 hours. The latent phase of dilatation is 6 hours compared with a normal mean of 4.8 but 13.6 hours is the maximum limit. The active phase of dilatation is almost 2 hours compared with a normal mean of 2.4 hours. A normal S curve is shown in the graph.

The descent pattern indicates a normal lack of engagement (about −1 to 0 station) before there is active labor. During the maximum slope of dilatation, the descent rate accelerates slowly and then very rapidly, bringing the presenting part to a visible point at the introitus. This is also indicative of a normal progression of labor.

Nothing in this graph indicates that other than routine labor care is warranted.

Patient B: Since the mean for labor of a nullipara is 11 hours, this 17-hour labor is slightly long. The mean of the latent phase of cervical dilatation is 6.4 hours (20.1 maximum); this latent phase is approximately 8 hours (12 Mn. to 8 A.M.) and therefore normal in length. The mean for the active phase of cervical dilatation is 4.6 hours (11.7 maximum); since the patient's active phase is 9 hours (8 A.M. to 5 P.M.), it is slightly longer than the mean. Two abnormalities in the active phase should be considered: the slow slope and arrest.

A slow slope in a nullipara is 1.2 cm or less dilatation per hour. From 8 A.M. to 4 P.M. (8 hours) this patient's cervix dilated 4½ cm (from 2 to 3 cm to 7 cm). Dilatation of 4½ cm in 8 hours is less than 1.2 cm per hour. This is the time when there is an abnormal progression in cervical dilatation for this patient.

Owing to soft tissue resistance in the pelvis, a slow slope frequently occurs in the nullipara. X-ray or ultrasound might be done if malposition or fetopelvic disproportion is suspected. Vaginal exams should be done as infrequently as possible. Because a stimulant is usually not helpful at this time, the best nursing intervention would be to provide comfort, relaxation, and support to the patient, since she is likely to become frustrated by the slow progress. Normal nursing observations of maternal and fetal conditions would be appropriate. Intravenous fluids should be given and the bladder frequently emptied. Analgesia/anesthesia could be given once in the active dilatation phase (following 4 cm dilatation).

Although there is no progress in cervical dilatation from 3 to 4 P.M., this does not meet the requirement of 2 hours for arrest in the active phase.

When analyzing the descent pattern of Patient B, it is apparent that the fetus is engaged (−1 to 0 station) at the onset of labor, which is normal for a nullipara. Little or no progression in descent until well into the active phase is normal. Acceleration in descent should take place during the maximum slope of dilatation, which it does. No special nursing interventions are therefore required.

CHAPTER **5**

NURSING CARE DURING LABOR STIMULATION

Janet S. Malinowski

In different areas of the country certain stimulants are used more than others. It is likely that the stimulants discussed in this chapter are not all inclusive, but they are the stimulants used most frequently.

OBJECTIVES

Upon completion of this chapter, the reader will be able to:

1. For the following stimulants—ambulation, enema, amniotomy, and oxytocin:
   a. explain the rationale for their stimulation of labor,
   b. discuss the nursing interventions appropriate before, during, and following stimulation,
   c. identify contraindications to their use.
2. Describe the effects that stripping the membranes and use of laminaria might have on the cervix.
3. Differentiate between surgical and medical induction.
4. Identify conditions that justify induction.
5. Apply the Bishop Scoring System to patient data and interpret the score.
6. Identify a drug being researched for labor induction.

LABOR STIMULANTS

Ambulation

Frequently a woman in false labor or early labor is advised to ambulate (walk) for 30 to 60 minutes or longer. Usually, ambulation causes false labor contractions to stop. These irregular contractions, although uncomfortable, cause minimal cervical changes. For the woman in early true labor, ambulation tends to stimulate uterine contractions. The upright position assumed when walking takes advantage of the principle of gravity and may encourage descent of the fetus. It also brings the fetus into a forward position so that the presenting fetal part is better aligned with the inlet of the pelvis. Pressure on the cervix by the presenting part may stimulate oxytocin production from the posterior pituitary; this in turn increases the frequency of contractions and causes progress in cervical dilatation.

When a woman is instructed to ambulate she needs to be told where she may go and when she should return. The instructions will depend on the hospital's facilities as well as her physical condition. If her membranes should rupture or the contractions become considerably more intense and frequent (2 to 3 minutes apart), she should be instructed to return to the unit immediately rather than to wait until the designated time. Providing someone to walk with her and informing her of the advantages of the activity usually result in more active walking. Periodic rests whether standing or sitting may be necessary and continue the positive effect of gravity's pressure. The nurse may need to provide a makeshift bathrobe and slippers so the woman will feel more presentable as she ambulates. Until the uterus is rhythmically contracting it is not necessary to retake a normal fetal heart rate more than every hour. When 1 to 3 hours of ambulation does not bring on true labor, discharge instructions should be given, including when to come back to the hospital. Undoubtedly the woman will be disappointed that she is not likely to have her baby that day, and she needs to be reassured that false alarms are not unusual.

Review Questions

1. What effect does ambulation usually have on false labor? _____

2. What response should a nurse have for a woman who experiences false labor? _____

_____

3. Identify three reasons why the upright position of ambulation may stimulate labor:
   a. _____
   b. _____
   c. _____

4. State four nursing interventions you would take upon receiving the order to ambulate a woman:
   a. _____
   b. _____
   c. _____
   d. _____

Answers

1. Ambulation usually stops false labor.

2. For a woman who experiences false labor, a nurse should provide discharge instructions about when to return to the hospital and provide reassurance that false labor is not uncommon.

3. The upright position a. encourages the fetus to gravitate (descend) in the pelvis. b. It brings the fetus into a forward position, aligning the fetus better with the inlet of the pelvis. c. It encourages the presenting part to press on the cervix, which may stimulate oxytocin production and thereby increase uterine contractions.

4. Upon receiving the order to ambulate a woman, the nurse should:
   a. Tell her why ambulation is desirable.
   b. Provide her with appropriate clothing, if necessary.
   c. Instruct her about where she can go and when she should return, including conditions that warrant early return.
   d. Provide someone to walk with her.
   e. Retake normal fetal heart rates approximately every hour.

Stripping Membranes

Many times a woman will come into the labor unit and say that her membranes were stripped in the doctor's office yesterday. Stripping the membranes involves inserting a digit (finger) through the uterine cervix and digitally loosening the membranes from the uterine wall in the region of the cervix. Stripping the membranes is appropriate when the uterine cervix is dilated sufficiently to permit entrance of a (doctor's) fingertip, and the presenting part is not above −1 station. This procedure sometimes initiates labor at term; it often encourages softening and effacement of the cervix. The woman often experiences cramping and slight vaginal bleeding following this procedure.

Review Questions

1. What is the purpose of stripping the membranes? _____
   _____

2. What physical effect might the woman experience following this procedure? _____

Answers

1. The purpose of stripping the membranes is to initiate labor and/or encourage softening and effacement of the cervix.
2. The woman might feel cramps and have slight vaginal bleeding.

Enemas

A Fleet or mild soapsuds enema is a stimulant frequently given to labor patients shortly after admission. There are strong arguments for giving an enema to a woman in early labor. 1. The intestinal peristalsis produced by the enema is transferred to the uterus and starts or enhances uterine contractions. 2. An enema efficiently empties a full rectum, providing more room for fetal descent through the birth canal. 3. A full rectum during Stage II of labor may result in defecation during the fetal expulsion phase, which will contaminate the introitus and/or sterile field at the time of delivery. 4. Defecation at this time might inhibit her willingness to push. However, in some hospitals an enema is routinely not given. The rationale is that an enema is uncomfortable and unnecessary, since the bowel will empty itself naturally prior to labor.

Before an enema is given, a brief patient history and vital signs, including the counting of a normal fetal heart rate (FHR), are taken and a vaginal examination is done. A woman in early labor with no abnormal vaginal bleeding and the fetal head well engaged is a likely candidate for an enema. Contraindications to giving an enema include:

1. vaginal bleeding suggestive of abruptio placentae (premature separation of the placenta) or placenta previa (the placenta implanted near the cervix) which may potentially cause profuse bleeding and place mother or fetus at risk for increased morbidity or mortality;

2. breech presentation, which increases the likelihood of prolapsed cord or spontaneous rupture of membranes due to the uneven fit of the buttocks or lower extremities in the pelvis;

3. premature labor, which decreases the chances of survival of the infant;

4. rupture of membranes (in some institutions), which increases the chances of infection as well as prolapsed cord if the head is not well engaged;

5. advanced labor (cervix dilated 6 cm or more), which stimulates labor to accelerate too rapidly.

A nurse can help a woman to cope with the enema procedure by finding out how much the woman knows and giving the necessary explanation. In the following ways the administration of a soapsuds enema to a woman in labor differs from those given to other adults:

1. the amount may be as much as 1500 to 2000 ml if tolerable;

2. the tubing is inserted up to 10 to 12 inches (the second mark on most tubes);

3. the air in the tubing does not need to be removed, since it tends to increase peristalsis;

4. during uterine contractions it may be necessary to clamp the tubing, give reassurance, and encourage the woman to concentrate on slow deep breathing techniques;

5. expulsion is immediate and requires approximately 20 minutes to complete;

6. the fetal heart rate is reassessed following the expulsion to assure that no significant changes have occurred.

Review Questions

1. Check (✓) the situations below that are contraindications to an enema:

   _____ abnormal or absent fetal heart rate

   _____ station − 2

   _____ vaginal bleeding (other than bloody show)

   _____ breech presentation

   _____ premature labor

   _____ rupture of membranes

   _____ cervix 7 cm dilated

2. When administering an enema what actions should the nurse take regarding the following?

   a. Fetal heart rate: _____

   _____

b. Amount of solution: _____

c. Insertion of tubing: _____

d. Complaint of discomfort during a contraction: _____

e. Expulsion of enema: _____

Answers

1. All of the situations given are contraindications to an enema, with the possible exception of rupture of membranes (depending on hospital protocol).

2. When administering an enema to a woman in labor the nurse should:
   a. Assess the fetal heart rate before giving the enema and immediately following the expulsion.
   b. Fill the bag with 1500 to 2000 ml of solution.
   c. Insert the tubing approximately 12 inches—to the second mark—without removing the air in the tubing.
   d. To decrease discomfort during a contraction have the woman breathe slowly and deeply, clamp tubing during the contraction, and provide necessary assurance.
   e. Provide for immediate expulsion, allowing at least 20 minutes for its completion.

Amniotomy

Another procedure that the doctor might perform to enhance labor is an amniotomy (commonly abbreviated AROM or ARM, meaning artificial rupture of the membranes). The procedure stimulates labor because the fetal head is then allowed to be in direct contact with the cervix. The fetal head is thought to be a better cervical dilating agent than the waters contained in the membranes.

Some authorities do not advise amniotomy early in labor. Caldeyro-Barcia and associates[1] found that there is an increased incidence of caput succedaneum (swelling of the fetal scalp), disalignment of the fetal cranial bones, and early decelerations in the fetal heart rate (not an ominous pattern). But they do advocate AROM when internal fetal monitoring is necessary; that is, in the presence of suspected fetal hypoxia and acidosis. Lynaugh[2] agrees that AROM should be reserved for when internal monitoring and fetal scalp pH determination are advisable. But he states that neonates have a good outcome following AROM despite the increased pressure on the fetal skull. He also found that AROM does not predictably shorten labor; when it does it is by a maximum of approximately one hour.

Despite the critics AROM is done frequently during early and mid-labor in hopes of shortening labor. When an amniotomy is performed the woman is placed on her back with her knees flexed. The fetal heart rate is taken just prior to AROM to assure fetal well-being at this time. After a sterile vaginal exam, the physician ruptures the amniotic sac with a sterile instrument: an amnihook (which resembles a crochet hook), an Allis forceps, or a 25-gauge needle. (Occasionally the membranes will accidentally be ruptured during vaginal exam.) In anticipation of the large amount of amniotic fluid that might be expelled, the nurse should place several absorbent pads under the woman's buttocks and inform her of a possible gush of warm fluid. No anesthesia is necessary for AROM for there are no nerve endings in the membranes. A small amount of blood from cervical trauma may be evident. If the procedure is explained before it is performed, the woman should be able to relax and experience no trauma.

Normally the fluid is light yellow or colorless, possibly cloudy. A dark color indicates fetal distress. (See Chapter 1.) The odor is normally nonoffensive. Foul smelling amniotic fluid is a sign of infection within the uterus. Since both the color and odor of the amniotic fluid are significant, they should be recorded on the woman's chart. In cases in which the amniotic sac ruptures spontaneously (abbreviated SROM or SRM), it may be necessary to ask the woman to describe the fluid, as well as to check the perineum or pads beneath the buttocks for the characteristics of the leaking amniotic fluid.

Doctors usually will not perform an AROM if the presenting part of the fetus is high (-2 or above) in the pelvis. When the amniotic sac is ruptured, the expulsion of fluid causes the presenting part to exert greater pressure on the cervix. If the cord is between the presenting part and the cervix, the cord may be pushed out (prolapsed) through the cervix or compressed between the fetal head and the cervix even though it may not be visible (an occult cord). In either case the fetal heart rate is abnormally slow. That is why it is imperative that the nurse take the fetal heart rate immediately after the membranes are ruptured.

Since all the amniotic fluid will not be expelled immediately, the woman should be told to expect to leak fluid, especially during contractions and when changing her position, until the time of birth when the fluid remaining in the top of the uterus and around the fetus will finally be expelled.

Review Questions

1. Why might AROM stimulate labor?_____
   _____

2. State four reasons why some authorities do not recommend AROM
   except when internal fetal monitoring is warranted:
   a. _____
   b. _____
   c. _____
   d. _____

3. What three measures should a nurse take before AROM is performed?
   a. _____
   b. _____
   c. _____

4. What three actions should a nurse perform immediately following
   AROM?
   a. _____
   b. _____
   c. _____

Answers

1. AROM stimulates labor by placing the fetal head in direct contact
   with the cervix; the head has a better dilating effect than the bag of
   waters.

2. Some authorities do not recommend AROM unless internal fetal
   monitoring is necessary, because there is an increased incidence in
   a. caput succedaneum; b. disalignment of the fetal cranial bones;
   and c. early decelerations of the fetal heart rate. d. AROM does not
   predictably shorten labor; when it does the maximum is by about
   one hour.

3. Before AROM is performed the nurse should:
   a.   Be certain that the fetal heart rate is normal.
   b.   Physically prepare the woman on her back with her knees bent
        and protection (padding) placed under her buttocks.
   c.   Explain to the woman what to expect: passage of warm fluid
        and a trickle of fluid from now until the baby is born.

4. Immediately following AROM the nurse should a. check and record
   the color and odor of the amniotic fluid; b. check for a prolapsed
   cord; and c. check and record the FHR for a normal pattern and
   rate.

Labor may accelerate following AROM, although this is not always the case. However, once the membranes are ruptured, additional precautions need to be taken. The intact amniotic sac served as a barrier against bacterial invasion. Once the membranes are ruptured, the fetus is open to infection. Therefore, vaginal exams should not be as frequent, since the examiner is a possible source of bacteria. The nurse will need to rely more on signs of progress other than cervical changes. (See Chapter 1.) Despite the stimulating effects of ambulation, it may increase exposure to bacteria. Therefore, in many hospitals the mother is confined to bed and instructed to use a bedpan for elimination. Since an increase in body temperature is a sign of infection, her temperature should be taken every 2 hours (every hour if elevated) following the rupture of membranes.

Most authorities believe that the fetus should be born within 24 hours after rupture of membranes. Some doctors strictly adhere to the 24-hour limit and will stimulate the labor by additional means (for example, oxytocin) if delivery is not imminent; or they will consider cesarean delivery; others will hold off for a day or two longer. Some doctors feel that as long as there is no apparent adverse effect on the woman or fetus, there is no need to deliver the fetus immediately. The woman might even be discharged from the hospital and sometimes be given a prescription for a prophylactic antibiotic. If she is discharged with ruptured membranes before delivery, the nurse should verify that the woman knows the signs of impending infection (increase in temperature, foul smelling and/or discolored amniotic fluid, rapid pulse) and how to get in touch with her doctor.

Review Questions

1.   Give four nursing measures that should be taken because of the increased likelihood of infection following rupture of membranes:
     a. _____
     b. _____
     c. _____
     d. _____

2.   If the woman asked you, "Will I have to deliver my baby within 24 hours, since my membranes are ruptured," how would you answer her? (Choose one.)
     a.   "Yes, doctors always deliver the baby within 24 hours after rupture of membranes."
     b.   "Yes, because infection may occur now that the barrier to infection—the membranes—has been broken."
     c.   "Not necessarily. It is desirable that you deliver within 24 hours, but we will watch you carefully. The status of you and your

baby and the progress of your labor will influence the doctor's decision if you have not delivered in 24 hours."

Answers

1. Nursing measures to be taken following rupture of membranes include:
   a. Take temperature at least every two hours.
   b. Watch for foul smelling, discolored amniotic fluid.
   c. Check for rapid pulse rate.
   d. Do vaginal exams as seldom as possible; rely on other signs of progress.
   e. Keep the woman in bed; offer bedpan as needed.

2. c is correct.

INDUCTION—A FORM OF LABOR STIMULATION

Ambulation and enema are classified as labor stimulants. They are not methods of induction. Rupture of membranes, a labor stimulant, is also a method of *surgical induction* of labor. The other form of induction is *medical induction,* which involves the use of medication; for example, oxytocin.

There are several advantages of induction. It may be planned ahead of time so the woman can enter labor well rested and psychologically prepared. There may be time to make the necessary arrangements for the household. The induction is usually planned for the day shift and on a weekday when the hospital is well staffed and equipped.

Prior to induction the woman should be required to sign a written consent form that lists and explains the most frequent complications and the frequency of their occurrences. These risks include prematurity, increased incidence of infection, postpartum hemorrhage, fetal distress, and failed induction.

For labor to be medically induced there must be specific indications. These include conditions in which continuation of pregnancy endangers the mother's health or the fetus' well-being. The following is a partial list of conditions warranting medical induction and the rationale for inducing labor:

1. prolonged rupture of membranes—to decrease the likelihood of infection, specifically amnionitis;

2. postmaturity—to prevent further fetal compromise (see Chapter 6);

3. maternal diabetes—to deliver 2 to 3 weeks preterm (based on fetal maturity studies) to prevent fetal demise due to placental insufficiency and to prevent growth beyond the size compatible with vaginal delivery;

4. pre-eclampsia or eclampsia—to reverse progression of the pregnancy-related condition,

5. Rh sensitization—to avert erythroblastosis fetalis (hemolytic disease) in the newborn involving CNS pathology due to high bilirubin level.

Before induction fetal maturity should be verified, since there is increased risk of fetal prematurity. Amniocentesis provides the L/S ratio and creatinine concentration. X-ray or ultrasound studies indicate the biparietal diameter (as well as adequacy of fetopelvic relationships). (See Chapter 6.)

Induction is usually not attempted unless the cervix is favorable—soft and beginning to efface and dilate—and the fetal head is presenting and engaged. The Bishop score is a method of assessing these factors and predicting readiness for induction. Scores range from 0 to 13. The higher the score is, the greater is the likelihood of successful induction of labor. A score of greater than 4 has an 80 percent success rate.[3] See Table 5-1.

In a situation in which the cervix is not ripe for induction, *laminaria tents* (sterile dried seaweed) occasionally may be placed within the cervix. As they absorb moisture they swell and may cause softening and dilatation of the cervix. Most of the swelling occurs in the first 6 hours with the maximum effect achieved in 24 hours.[4] Another more controversial method is prostaglandin E_2 (PGE$_2$). This is a viscous gel suppository which is inserted in the cervix and has been experimentally effective in producing rapid and prominent cervical ripening.[5,6] When laminaria or prostaglandin is used, oxytocin infusion is frequently necessary to achieve true labor.

TABLE 5-1 Bishop Score*

| | ASSIGNED VALUE | | | |
FACTOR	0	1	2	3
Cervical dilatation	Closed	1–2 cm	3–4 cm	5 cm or more
Cervical effacement	0–30%	40–50%	60–70%	80% or more
Fetal station	−3	−2	−1, 0	+1, +2
Cervical consistency	Firm	Moderate	Soft	
Cervical position	Posterior	Midposition	Anterior	

*Modified from: BISHOP, EH: *Pelvic scoring for elective induction.* Obstet Gynecol 24:266, 1964.

Review Questions

1. Fill in the blanks:
   a. Rupture of membranes is called _____ induction.
   b. The use of oxytocin is called _____ induction.
   c. Labor induced because mother or fetus would be jeopardized by continuation of the pregnancy is called _____ induction.

2. What are some advantages of induction?
   a. _____
   b. _____
   c. _____

3. What conditions justify medically indicated induction?
   a. _____
   b. _____
   c. _____

4. Why might amniocentesis and x-ray or ultrasound be done before induction is begun? _____
   _____
   _____

5. What information does a Bishop score of greater than 4 provide?
   _____
   _____
   _____

6. Why would laminaria be placed in the cervix for up to 24 hours?
   _____
   _____
   _____

Answers

1. a. Rupture of membranes is called *surgical* induction.
   b. The use of oxytocin is called *medical* induction.
   c. Labor induced because mother or fetus would be jeopardized by continuation of the pregnancy is called *medically indicated* induction.

2. Advantages of induction include a. planned time for labor; b. mother rested; c. mother psychologically prepared for labor; d. necessary household arrangements made; and e. hospital usually well staffed and equipped.

3. Conditions that justify indicated induction include a. prolonged rupture of membranes; b. postmaturity; c. maternal diabetes; d. pre-eclampsia/eclampsia; and e. Rh sensitization.

4. Amniocentesis and x-ray or ultrasound may be done before induction is begun to verify fetal maturity. X-ray or ultrasound may also be done to ascertain pelvic adequacy.

5. Based on the status of the cervix and fetal station, a Bishop score of greater than 4 predicts that there is an 80 percent chance of success in induction of labor at this time.

6. Laminaria is dried seaweed that, when placed in the cervix, absorbs moisture and may cause the cervix to soften and dilate. It reaches its maximum effect by 24 hours.

Induction of Labor with Oxytocin

Oxytocin is the drug used most frequently for medical induction of labor. (It is also used for *augmentation*—to improve or reinforce labor; for example, in hypotonic uterine contractions.) As the pregnancy approaches term the uterus becomes very sensitive to minute amounts of oxytocin. Natural oxytocin eventually is released from the posterior lobe of the pituitary gland and stimulates rhythmic uterine contractions. Synthetic preparations of oxytocin (for example, Pitocin and Syntocinon) likewise act on the smooth muscle of the uterus to stimulate contractions. These contractions are often more painful than noninduced contractions owing to their comparatively rapid onset. (Ergots, another classification of oxytocics which includes Methergine, cause sustained uterine contractions that are incompatible with adequate fetal oxygenation and therefore should not be used until following delivery.)

CONTRAINDICATIONS TO INDUCTION WITH OXYTOCIN. Induction should not be done in the presence of abnormal fetopelvic relationships. These include fetopelvic disproportion, malpresentation, and malposition. Nor should labor be induced when the fetal status is already in jeopardy; for example, in the presence of fetal distress or prematurity. In the presence of uterine scar tissue or hypertonic uterine contractions, induction is likely to result in uterine rupture. Induction with oxytocin would cause increased risk to mother and fetus in the presence of severe pre-eclampsia and placenta previa.

Review Question

Reread the previous paragraph. Underline the 9 specific conditions that are contraindications to induction with oxytocin.

Answers

1. fetopelvic disproportion; 2. malpresentation; 3. malposition; 4. fetal distress; 5. prematurity; 6. uterine scar tissue; 7. hypertonic uterine contractions; 8. severe pre-eclampsia; and 9. placenta previa.

THE ADMINISTRATION OF OXYTOCIN INDUCTION. Oxytocin is always administered intravenously. An infusion pump is preferred, since it precisely controls the amount of medicine administered. A piggyback setup—two IV bottles of the same solution, one with oxytocin and one without—makes it possible to discontinue the oxytocin immediately if necessary without disturbing the intravenous infusion. Ten units (10,000 mU) of oxytocin are placed in 1000 ml of 5% dextrose in water or lactated Ringer's solution. The initial dose may be as low as 0.5 but not more than 2 mU per minute. At 15- to 20-minute intervals the rate is increased by no more than 1 to 2 mU per minute until a normal uterine contraction pattern begins. Oxytocin must be administered with extreme caution because its effect is unpredictable. Ideally the contractions will attain a frequency of 2 to 3 minutes, a duration of 45 to 60 seconds, and an intensity of moderate to strong with at least a 30-second resting period.

A qualified physician must remain on the labor unit whenever oxytocin is being administered. The physician or nurse must assess the uterine contractions and fetal response at least every 15 minutes. An external or internal electronic monitor is routinely in place. The oxytocin dose should be recorded on the monitor's graph paper each time the dose is altered. Tetanic contractions (lasting longer than 90 seconds) and tumultuous (violently agitated) labor may result and cause 1. fetal distress due to impaired placental and fetal circulation during the contractions; 2. abruptio placentae (premature separation of the placenta); 3. amniotic fluid emboli; 4. lacerations to the cervix and neonatal injuries; and 5. rupture of the uterus. In the presence of any of the above complications, the oxytocin must be discontinued immediately and the doctor must be informed. The half-life of oxytocin is 3 to 4 minutes; therefore its discontinuance may get rapid results.

While oxytocin is being given it is the nurse's responsibility to check and report urine output, as well as to monitor vital signs. Prolonged use of oxytocin can cause water intoxication (antidiuresis). A high concentration of oxytocin may cause hypertension accompanied by a frontal headache; both of these side effects disappear when the drug is stopped.

If the desired labor does not occur within 8 hours the oxytocin is discontinued and the other solution in the piggyback is infused at a keep-open rate. On a second day, or even a third, induction may be tried again, depending on the status of the mother and fetus.

Review Questions

1. What are the actions of oxytocin? _____
   _____

2. Name two oxytocics used to stimulate labor:
   a. _____   b. _____

3. Summarize the nursing interventions appropriate during the administration of oxytocin:
   a. Set up piggyback IV of: _____
      _____
   b. Give initial rate of: _____
   c. Increase rate every _____ by (what
      amount?) _____ depending on: _____
      _____
   d. Assess uterine contractions and fetal heart rate every:
      _____
   e. Maintain rate that causes ideal contractions, which are:
      _____
      _____
   f. Stop the induction immediately in the presence of _____
      contractions or _____ labor.
   g. Monitor vital signs for _____ and I&O for
      _____
   h. If the first day of induction is not successful, prepare mother
      for: _____
      _____

Answers

1. Oxytocin stimulates rhythmic uterine contractions.

2. a. Pitocin and b. Syntocinon are oxytocics used to stimulate labor.

3. Nursing interventions appropriate during administration of oxytocin:
   a. Set up piggyback IV of one bottle with 1000 ml 5% D/W or RL
      and a second bottle with the same solution but with 10 U
      oxytocin added.
   b. Give initial rate of 0.5 to 2 mU per minute.
   c. Increase rate every *15 to 20 minutes* by *1 to 2 mU per min
      intervals,* depending on uterine response and fetal heart rate.
   d. Assess uterine contractions and fetal heart rate *every 15
      minutes.*

e.   Maintain rate that causes ideal contractions, which are every 2 to 3 minutes, 45 to 60 seconds duration, of moderate to strong intensity, with at least a 30-second rest period.

f.   Stop the induction immediately in the presence of *tetanic* contractions or *tumultuous* labor.

g.   Monitor vital signs for *hypertension* and I&O for *signs of water intoxication.*

h.   If the first day of induction is not successful, prepare the mother for a possible second or third day of induction.

Induction of Labor with Prostaglandin

Prostaglandin in numerous forms continues to be researched as an agent to induce labor at or near term. Among the distressing side effects of prostaglandin are the frequent occurrence of uterine hypertonicity and gastrointestinal upset (nausea, vomiting, diarrhea). Prostaglandin is available and is used abroad but currently is not approved for use during labor in the United States.

CONCLUSION

Stimulation of labor has gained much favor in our fast moving, highly technological society. Stimulation has merit when used judiciously. Nurses can help to make the use of labor stimulants more acceptable to pregnant women and their families by providing information and supportive care before and during the labor stimulation process.

REFERENCES

1.   CALDEYRO-BARCIA, R, ET AL: *Adverse perinatal effects of early amniotomy during labor.* In GLUCK, B (ED): *Modern Perinatal Medicine.* Year Book Medical Publishers, Chicago, 1974, pp 431–449.

2.   LYNAUGH, KH: *The effects of early elective amniotomy on the length of labor and the condition of the fetus.* J Nurs-Midw 25:3, 1980.

3.   FRIEDMAN, EA: *Labor: Clinical Evaluation and Management.* Appleton-Century-Crofts, New York, 1978, p 334.

4.   OXORN, H: *Human Labor and Birth.* Appleton-Century-Crofts, New York, 1980, p 589.

5.   ULMSTEN, U: *Aspects of ripening the cervix and induction of labor by intra-cervical application of PGE_2 in viscous gel.* Acta Obstet Gynecol Scand (Suppl) 84:5, 1979.

6.   STEINER, H, ET AL: *Cervical ripening prior to induction of labor.* Prostaglandins 17:125, 1979.

BIBLIOGRAPHY

BENSON, RC: *Current Obstetric and Gynecologic Diagnosis and Treatment,* ed 3. Lange Medical Publications, Los Altos, Calif., 1980.

CALDEYRO-BARCIA, R, ET AL: *Adverse perinatal effects of early amniotomy during labor.* In GLUCK, L (ED): *Modern Perinatal Medicine.* Year Book Medical Publisher, Chicago, 1974.

DHEW: *New Restrictions on Oxytocin Use.* FDA Drug Bulletin 8(5):30, 1978.

FRIEDMAN, EA: *Labor: Clinical Evaluation and Management,* ed 2. Appleton-Century-Crofts, New York, 1978.

HAWKINS, JW AND HIGGINS, LP: *Maternity and Gynecological Nursing: Women's Health Care.* JB Lippincott, Philadelphia, 1981.

JOHNSON, GG: *Oxytocics for the Induction of Labor.* In Series 3 *IntraPartal Care Module.* March of Dimes Birth Defects Foundation, White Plains, NY, 1981.

KOZIER, B AND ERB, GL: *Fundamentals of Nursing: Concepts and Procedures.* Addison-Wesley, Menlo Park, Calif., 1979, pp 624–27.

LYNAUGH, KH: *The effects of early elective amniotomy on the length of labor and the condition of the fetus.* J N-Midw 25(4):3, 1980.

NAACOG: *Induction of Labor.* NAACOG Technical Bulletin #4, 1979.

OLDS, SB, ET AL: *Obstetric Nursing.* Addison-Wesley, Menlo Park, Calif., 1980.

OXORN, H: *Human Labor and Birth,* ed 4. Appleton-Century-Crofts, New York, 1980.

QUILLIGAN, EJ AND KRETCHMER, N: *Fetal and Maternal Medicine.* John Wiley & Sons, New York, 1980.

ROBERTS, J.: *Alternate positions for childbirth—Part I: First stage of labor.* J Nurs-Midw 25(4):11, 1980.

ROSENBERG, LS, ET AL: *Preinduction ripening of the cervix with laminaria in the nulliparous patient.* J Reprod Med 25(2):60, 1980.

STEINER, H, ET AL: *Cervical ripening prior to induction of labor.* Prostaglandins 17(1):125, 1979.

TOHAN, N, ET AL: *Ripening of the term cervix with laminaria.* Obstet Gynecol 54(5):588, 1979.

ULMSTEN, U: *Aspects of ripening the cervix and induction of labor by intracervical application of PGE_2 in viscous gel.* Acta Obstet Gynecol Scand (Suppl) 84:5, 1979.

POST-TEST

1. An enema is given to a labor patient because it: (Circle True or False).
    a. T F   might stimulate uterine contractions.
    b. T F   empties the lower intestinal tract.
    c. T F   prevents the likelihood of fecal contamination during delivery.

d.   T   F   may cause less inhibition to push following complete cervical dilatation.

2.   In which of the following situations should a nurse question the order for an enema for a labor patient? (Circle yes or no)
   a.   Y   N   Patient is bleeding in excess of bloody show.
   b.   Y   N   A primigravida's cervix is 3 cm dilated and station is -2.
   c.   Y   N   A multipara's cervix is 3 cm dilated and station is 0.
   d.   Y   N   The fetus is in breech presentation.
   e.   Y   N   The fetus is post-term.

3.   When giving an enema to a tense patient in early labor, what information about the procedure can you give the patient that might ease the situation? (Include at least 4 suggestions.)

_____

_____

_____

_____

4.   Circle True or False and explain your answer.
   a.   T   F   Stripping the membranes and rupture of membranes are the same thing.
   b.   T   F   Ambulation is contraindicated once labor begins.
   c.   T   F   As the laminaria swells it may cause progress in cervical changes.

5.   Explain why:
   a.   Fetal heart rate should be taken immediately following AROM.

_____

_____

   b.   The presence of dark-colored, foul smelling fluid is significant in a vertex presentation.

_____

_____

   c.   A woman with ruptured membranes is usually confined to bed.

_____

_____

6.   Which of the following responses are correct? Pitocin and Syntocinon:
   a.   are forms of oxytocin.
   b.   stimulate labor if the cervix is ripe.
   c.   may cause water intoxication (antidiuresis).
   d.   may alter the fetal heart rate and the maternal blood pressure.
   e.   require observation for uterine hypertonicity.

7. Which of the following principles should be observed in the use of oxytocin to stimulate labor?
   a. The condition of the fetus must be satisfactory.
   b. Oxytocin should be used only in cases of uterine dysfunction.
   c. There must be no predisposition to uterine rupture.
   d. Oxytocin should be used in cases in which it is important to terminate the pregnancy quickly, e.g., in abruptio placentae.
   e. A responsible physician should be constantly available while the mother is receiving oxytocin.
8. Mrs. Adam, a G3 P2, is 41 weeks pregnant. Her cervix is dilated 2 cm, soft, 20 percent effaced, anterior. The fetal station is − 2. Using the Bishop scoring system, interpret her chances for being successfully induced.

   _____
   _____
   _____
   _____
   _____

9. The name of a type of experimental labor induction drug is _____
   _____ .

Answers

1. a. True; b. True; c. True; and d. True.
2. a. yes; b. yes; c. no; d. yes; and e. no.
3. To ease the situation while giving a tense patient an enema:
   a. familiarize the patient with the equipment, inform her of the length of time she will need to retain the solution, and tell her that she will be allowed to completely evacuate the contents on the toilet.
   b. inform her that: the procedure should not hurt, the tube will be lubricated, and if resistance is met, the tube will be stopped and repositioned; the procedure can be stopped during contractions.
   c. inform her that the flow of solution can be stopped when she feels enough pressure and/or uterine contractions occur.
   d. tell the patient to try slow deep breathing during the procedure.
   e. explain the purposes for the enema (see Question 1).
4. a. False. Stripping of membranes is a digital loosening of the membranes from the uterus and is done to encourage cervical softening and effacement. Rupture of membranes involves breaking the membranes.

b. False. Ambulation may be encouraged during early labor, since it may stimulate labor. (There are some instances when it is contraindicated, for example, following ROM or sedation.)

c. True. Laminaria absorbs moisture from the cervix, causing the laminaria to swell and possibly causing the cervix to soften and dilate.

5. a. An abnormal fetal heart rate pattern may indicate abnormal pressure on the cord. This may occur following AROM.

b. Dark-colored amniotic fluid indicates meconium, which is abnormal in vertex presentation. A foul smell indicates possible infection.

c. The woman is confined to bed to reduce the chance of introducing infection.

6. All of the responses about Pitocin and Syntocinon are correct.

7. a, c, and e are correct.

8. The Bishop scoring system gives Mrs. Adam a total of 6 points: 1 point for 2 cm, 2 for soft, 0 for 20 percent, 1 for -2 station, 2 for anterior. A score greater than 4 gives her a success rate of 80 percent. (She also has in her favor a term pregnancy and probably nonresistent pelvic soft tissue, since she is a multipara.)

9. *Prostaglandin* is the name of a type of experimental labor induction drug.

CHAPTER 6

CARING FOR WOMEN EXPERIENCING PREMATURE AND POST-TERM LABORS

Janet S. Malinowski

Delivery within two weeks of the predetermined due date is an expectation that both a pregnant woman and health professionals have. Premature labor, before 38 weeks gestation, may start spontaneously or may be medically induced (started). There is a significant increase in morbidity and mortality when labor occurs before 38 weeks, as well as when labor has not occurred by 42 weeks (post-term). This chapter deals with the reasons for concern and the interventions that can be used for premature and post-term labors. The nurse plays a key role in providing information, emotional support, and physical care in these situations.

OBJECTIVES

Upon completion of this chapter, the reader will be able to:

1. Define preterm and post-term in relation to gestational age.
2. Relate three psychologic effects that a premature labor or a post-term labor are likely to have on a woman.
3. Specify four physiologic handicaps that occur in the preterm infant and four in the post-term infant.
4. Explain and interpret at least four methods nurses use to determine the gestational age of a fetus.
5. Compare physical features of a preterm infant with those of a postmature infant.

continued on next page

6. Describe the nursing interventions involved in the following tests: amniocentesis, 24-hour urine for estriol, nonstress test, Oxytocin Challenge Test.
7. State the nursing implications of administering betamethasone, ritodrine, terbutaline, Vasodilan, and ethyl alcohol.
8. State five nursing measures to be instituted when premature delivery is imminent.
9. Identify four psychologic tasks of mothers of preterm infants.
10. Discuss four ways that a nurse can facilitate parental-infant attachment following a premature birth.
11. Identify appropriate nursing interventions to be used during post-term labor.
12. Identify the immediate care needed following delivery, based on the physiologic handicaps of the postmature infant.

PREMATURE LABOR

Psychologic Effects of Premature Labor on the Mother

Pregnancy is a time for maturation of the fetus as well as of the mother. Forty weeks, plus or minus two, are required for this to occur. If the fetus is delivered before this time, the chances of survival are decreased because it is physically immature. If the mother delivers before 38 weeks, she may not have had sufficient time to physically and mentally prepare for her new role. It is during the last trimester that the mother begins to *nest*— to prepare the house and the family for the new baby. It is the time when she begins to *let go* of those habits and activities that are incompatible with caring for a new baby. Around the seventh month of pregnancy, she begins to think about possibly losing and hurting the fetus. This is apparent in overprotective shielding of self. As her due date approaches these fears begin to subside. She actively wishes for termination of the pregnancy, to separate from the fetus, to end the symbiotic relationship between mother and fetus. By the last few weeks of a full-term pregnancy, she is physically uncomfortable owing to her large-sized abdomen, clumsiness, and fatigue.

The woman who goes into premature labor may not have completed the preparatory processes. She may not be ready to break the close relationship that only she has with the fetus. The result is that she may not be ready to take on the role of a mother as quickly or as easily as a woman who has carried her baby to term. She is also justified in being concerned about whether or not her preterm baby will survive.

Review Question

State three ways in which a woman who experiences a premature labor may not psychologically be prepared for her baby.

a. _____

b. _____

c. _____

Answers

Psychologically a woman may not be prepared for premature labor because:

a.   she may not have completed nesting—preparing the household for the baby.

b.   she may not have let go of the things in her life that are incompatible with caring for a new baby.

c.   she may have great fears of losing or hurting her baby, especially in the seventh month of pregnancy.

d.   she may wish to continue to carry her baby in utero rather than to be separated from a fetus that has become so much a part of her.

Physiologic Handicaps of the Preterm Infant

A baby born prematurely (having a gestational age of less than 38 weeks) is called *preterm*. The closer he is to term gestation, the better are his chances of survival. For many reasons the preterm infant has difficulty maintaining physiologic homeostasis and therefore is constantly threatened by any form of stress.

Preterm infants are hindered by difficult respirations. The center of the brain controlling respirations is poorly developed. The intercostal muscles and soft thoracic cage are weak. The involved capillaries are few in number and oxygen utilization is inefficient due to insufficient surfactant (which decreases surface tension) in the alveoli.

They have poor control of their body temperature owing to poor peripheral circulation, little fatty insulation, and low heat production.

They experience a disturbance in the intake and utilization of food. They tire easily and have a weak suck. Their stomach capacity is small and the existing enzymes are insufficient for complete digestion and absorption.

They are unable to handle infections adequately. They have thin, fragile skin and mucous membranes that are poor barriers against infection. They have a low level of antibodies circulating in the plasma (immunoglobins), immature phagocytosis, and an inability to localize infection.

They have a tendency towards anemia and hemorrhage. Their thin, fragile capillaries are easily damaged. Their slow response to vitamin K_1 further complicates their rapidly falling hemoglobin level and decreased coagulation factors.

They are also handicapped by a tendency towards fluid-electrolyte imbalance due to an inability to excrete sodium and chloride and to concentrate urine, as well as inadequate stores of glycogen and calcium.

These facts are presented so that you will better appreciate the need for sound medical judgment in determining whether or not the fetus is mature enough to be delivered.

Review Question

List 4 physiologic handicaps found in the preterm infant.

a. _____

b. _____

c. _____

d. _____

Answers

A preterm infant has the following physiologic handicaps:
   a.   Respirations are difficult and inefficient.
   b.   Body temperature is poorly controlled.
   c.   Intake and utilization of food is disturbed—poor intake, poor use.
   d.   Response to infection is poor.
   e.   A strong tendency towards anemia and hemorrhage exists.
   f.   Fluid and electrolytes are unbalanced; the premature infant is unable to excrete, concentrate, and store them adequately.

Methods of Determining Gestational Age

During routine antepartum care several techniques are performed by the nurse or doctor to approximate the gestational age.

1. The *EDC* (estimated date of confinement or delivery) is determined by using Naegele's rule; subtract 3 months and add 7 days and one year to the date of onset of the woman's last menstrual period (LMP).

EXAMPLE: LMP = 5/10/83; EDC = 2/17/84

There are 40 weeks between 5/10/83 and 2/17/84.

2. The time of *quickening* (the woman's first perception of fetal movement) is determined. This usually occurs at 16 to 18 weeks but may be confused with intestinal activity.

3. Using an ultrasonic device (for example, a Doppler) a *fetal heart rate* (FHR) can first be determined about 10 to 12 weeks; with a fetoscope an FHR can first be demonstrated at 18 to 20 weeks.

4. The *fundal height* is measured from the upper border of the symphysis pubis to the top of the fundus. The fundus is usually midway between the symphysis pubis and umbilicus at 16 weeks. At 20 weeks the fundus is at or just below the umbilicus. After 20 weeks, the number of weeks gestation is equal to the fundal height in cm, plus or minus 2 cm (for example, 24 weeks = 22 to 26 cm). At 24 weeks the fundus is just above the umbilicus. A uterus larger than expected is significant because it may be due to multiple gestation, hydatidiform mole, hydramnios, or maternal diabetes. A large uterus could also indicate a large but healthy fetus. Conversely, a smaller-than-expected uterus may indicate intrauterine growth retardation (IUGR). IUGR may be associated with chronic intrauterine insufficiency, a fetal anomaly, or a normal, small-size fetus.

Further diagnostic measures (ultrasound, x-ray, amniocentesis) may be necessary if there is uncertainty about the gestational period. *Ultrasound* (U/S), done in the x-ray department, transmits a photographable view of the *biparietal diameter* (BPD) of the fetal head and the *crown-rump length*. Beginning in the 13th week of gestation by doing serial measurements at least 2 to 3 weeks apart, the amount of fetal growth can be traced. The astute technician or nurse will use the opportunity to point out the placenta and umbilical cord, explaining their functions. By seeing her baby's image, the mother's fantasy of the baby becomes a reality. A full bladder is necessary during the procedure so that the relationship of other structures, especially the placenta, can be assessed. The bladder may cause some discomfort; however, the U/S procedure is painless. Less frequently, *x-rays* are done to determine bony landmarks and ossification centers; the distal femoral epiphysis is visible at 37 weeks. Ultrasound and x-ray help to determine fetal weight and growth.

The purpose of *amniocentesis* is to obtain laboratory specimens that indicate fetal maturity. The specimens are assessed for L/S ratio, foam, creatinine, and fat cells (to name the most common). Prior to the removal of amniotic fluid from the uterine cavity, the procedure needs to be explained to the mother, and a patient consent form should be signed. There is approximately 1 percent risk of spontaneous abortion, premature labor, trauma to fetus or placenta, and infection. The nurse should check the fetal heart rate just before and immediately after the procedure, and two hours later. In order to prevent penetration of the placenta with the needle, the placenta may be localized via U/S, or the physician may abdominally palpate the fetal position and then estimate the placental position by auscultating the uterine souffle (sounds of blood in uterine arteries). To avoid supine hypotension during the procedure, the mother lies on her side propped with pillows or with her head and shoulders slightly elevated. The nurse cleanses the abdomen with antiseptic (Betadine) solution using sterile technique. Local anesthetic is sometimes used at the site of entry into the abdomen, although the discomfort is slight; that is, comparable with that of having blood drawn. With a long 20- to 22-gauge needle 20 to 50 ml of amniotic fluid is removed by the doctor. The Betadine solution is removed with pHisoHex and water, the area dried, and the insertion site covered with a bandage. The amniotic fluid is sent to the laboratory for the following possible fetal maturity studies:

1. The *L/S ratio* can predict fetal lung maturity. When lechithin (L factor) exceeds sphingomyelin (S factor) by 2:1 or greater—usually by 35 to 36 weeks gestation—fetal pulmonary maturity and function are compatible with extrauterine life. With a 2:1 ratio there is enough *surfactant* (made up chiefly of lechithin) secreted by the fetal lungs to facilitate pulmonary gas exchange at the time of extrauterine breathing. An exception is the infant of a diabetic mother, in which case a 2:1 ratio does not assure lung maturity. The *foam test* is a simple, rapid test for lung maturity but is less precise than the L/S ratio. By mixing 1 part 90% ethanol with 2 parts amniotic fluid in a test tube, foam (bubbles) appears on the surface. If 15 minutes later a complete ring of foam remains, lung maturity is assumed. False-positive results are possible.

2. *Creatinine,* which indicates increased fetal muscle mass, is secreted by the fetal kidneys into the amniotic fluid. By at least 37 weeks gestation there are 2 mg creatinine per 100 ml of amniotic fluid. This is an indirect measurement of pulmonary maturity and can be affected by complications such as IUGR.

3. *Fat cells* from the fetal skin are also found in amniotic fluid. If more than 20 percent of the fluid is fat cells, the gestational age is thought to be 36 weeks or more.

4. The surfactant phospholipids are measured in the process of doing a lung profile on the amniotic fluid. One of these lipids is phosphatidyl glycerol (PG), which is a lung stabilizer. In the infant of an insulin-dependent diabetic mother, when PG is present and the L/S ratio is 2:1 or greater, there is greater accuracy in the diagnosis of lung maturity. Without PG there is an increased incidence of neonatal lung immaturity and hypoglycemia and excessive fetal growth.

Review Questions

1.   Methods of determining gestational age are listed in the chart below.

Hypothetical findings are given. Fill in the third column with your estimate of the gestational age.

ESTIMATING GESTATIONAL AGE

Method	Finding	Estimate of Gestational Age
a. EDC compared with today's date	a. Premature	a.
b. Quickening	b. Experienced 4 weeks ago	b.
c. Fetal heart rate	c. Not audible by fetoscope, but audible by Doppler	c.
d. Fundal weight	d. 27 cm	d.
e. Amniotic fluid via amniocentesis: 1a. L/S ratio 1b. Foam test 2. Creatinine 3. Fat cells	e. 1a. 2:1 1b. 15 min later, foam ring present 2. 2 mg/100 ml fluid 3. more than 20%	e. 1a. 1b. 2. 3.

2. List at least 5 nursing interventions to be taken during an amniocentesis:
   a.
   b.
   c.
   d.
   e.

Answers

1. a. Prematurity is *less than 38 weeks* gestation.
   b. If quickening occurred 4 weeks ago, gestation is *20 to 22 weeks*.
   c. A fetal heart rate not audible by fetoscope indicates *less than 18 to 20 weeks* gestation, but audible by Doppler indicates *at least 10 to 12 weeks*.
   d. Fundal height of 27 cm indicates *approximately 27 weeks* gestation.
   e. 1a. An L/S ratio of 2:1 indicates *35 + weeks gestation*.
   e. 1b. The presence of a foam ring after 15 minutes during a foam test indicates the *lungs may be mature*.

e. 2. 2 mg creatinine in 100 ml of fluid indicates *at least 37 weeks gestation.*

e. 3. Fat cells more than 20 percent indicates *36 weeks or more gestation.*

2. Nursing interventions during an amniocentesis include:
   a. Determine mother's understanding of the procedure and its purpose.
   b. Verify that a patient consent form has been signed.
   c. Check fetal heart rate before, immediately after, and 2 hours following the procedure.
   d. Position mother on her side with head and shoulders slightly elevated.
   e. Cleanse abdomen with antiseptic solution using sterile technique.
   f. Provide support to the mother as needed.
   g. Remove Betadine with pHisoHex and water, air dry, and apply bandage following completion of procedure.

Interventions to Arrest Premature Labor

Although premature labor often is associated with conditions such as abruptio placentae, premature rupture of membranes, an overdistended uterus, or poor nutrition, the triggering factor is still unknown. Sometimes uterine contractions, once begun, decrease spontaneously. Nonspecific measures that may reduce uterine activity are 1. bed rest in a lying-down position (which decreases hydrostatic forces on the cervix); and 2. hydration with IV and oral fluids (which indirectly inhibits hormonal stimulation of uterine contractions).

Tocolytic agents (drugs that arrest premature labor) should be considered if the following criteria exist: a live fetus, intact membranes, a cervix dilated less than 4 cm, no medical or obstetric contraindications, and no intrauterine infection. Exceptions may be made; for example, labor may be inhibited for a few days in the presence of rupture of membranes, although the risk of infection exists. This is especially true in the presence of fetal lung immaturity.

When the gestational period is less than 32 weeks, *betamethasone* (Celestone) may be given to the mother (6 to 12 mg IM every 12 to 24 hours × 2). It may be effective in accelerating lung maturity if delivery does not occur prior to 48 hours following the first injection. Contraindications to this drug include pre-eclampsia, diabetes, infection, and placental insufficiency. Betamethasone may stimulate maternal pulmonary edema.

Several *beta-mimetic* drugs, ritodrine, terbutaline, and isoxsuprine, are used as tocolytic agents. This group of drugs stimulates the beta

156   NURSING CARE OF THE LABOR PATIENT receptors in the myometrium and thereby inhibits uterine contractions. Nursing responsibilities during the administration of any of these drugs are similar.

Ritodrine (Yutopar) causes significant uterine inhibition and has only a few mild side effects. The most significant is maternal tachycardia (greater than 140 BPM) which requires reduction in the infusion rate. Although ritodrine is contraindicated in the presence of several conditions (for example, hemorrhage, uncontrolled diabetes, and severe preeclampsia), these contraindications are clearly identified in the literature. Ritodrine given with or without corticosteroids (for example, betamethasone) places the woman at risk for pulmonary edema.

Given via IV infusion pump according to hospital protocol, ritodrine is increased until the uterine contractions stop; then infusion is maintained at that rate for approximately 12 hours. Thirty to 60 minutes prior to stopping the IV infusion, oral therapy of ritodrine is begun. The woman is maintained on small doses until 38 weeks gestation. If preterm labor recurs, IV infusion can be restarted immediately.

During the IV administration the woman is kept in a left lateral position with her head elevated to prevent hypotension and facilitate placental perfusion. External electronic monitors are used to assess uterine contractions and fetal tachycardia or decreased baseline variability. Until the blood pressure, pulse, and fetal heart rate are stable, they should be assessed and recorded at least every 15 minutes. The woman's state of hydration also needs to be monitored.

Terbutaline (Bricanyl, Brethine) is another tocolytic agent that is administered IV by infusion pump. Although it frequently causes maternal and fetal tachycardia, the maternal blood pressure remains relatively stable. Nervousness, tremors, palpitations, and dizziness are common side effects. Maternal pulmonary congestion is again a potential complication when combined with corticosteroid therapy. Frequent assessment of contractions, fetal heart rate, and maternal vital signs is necessary throughout the IV therapy. Upon cessation of contractions, intramuscular subcutaneous, or oral therapy is used; vital signs should be monitored prior to each dose and 1 to 2 hours after.

Isoxsuprine (Vasodilan) also decreases uterine contractions by the beta-mimetic method and is most effective when given intravenously. Upon cessation of contractions for 12 to 24 hours, the route of administration is changed to IM and then oral. In addition to often causing maternal tachycardia and hypotension and fetal tachycardia, Vasodilan produces drowsiness, nervousness, and sweating. Although the contractions become less frequent, they often become stronger. Because of the frequent incidence of these side effects, Vasodilan is no longer the beta-mimetic drug of choice in most situations.

Review Questions

1. What are two nonspecific measures to reduce uterine activity?
   a. _____   b. _____

2. Betamethasone is given to _____

3. During the administration of ritodrine, terbutaline, and isoxsuprine, similar nursing interventions are appropriate. Identify five of them.
   a. _____   d. _____
   b. _____   e. _____
   c. _____

Answers

1. The nonspecific measures to reduce uterine activity are a. *bed rest in a lying-down position;* and b. *hydration with oral and IV fluids.*

2. Betamethasone is given to *accelerate fetal lung maturity.*

3. During the administration of ritodrine, terbutaline, and isoxsuprine, the following nursing interventions are appropriate:
   a. Confine the mother to bed; have her assume a (side) lying position.
   b. Monitor uterine contraction status.
   c. Monitor fetal heart rate—specifically watch for tachycardia and decreased baseline variability.
   d. Monitor blood pressure for hypotension and pulse for tachycardia.
   e. Increase IV rate gradually (according to hospital protocol) if uterine contractions continue.
   f. Assess for maternal pulmonary edema.
   g. Continue medication by other than IV route following cessation of contractions.

For many years alcohol was, and in some places still is, used to arrest premature labor. *Ethyl alcohol* arrests labor by inhibiting the release of oxytocin (which is thought to play a dominant role in the initiation and maintenance of labor). It is administered intravenously. A very large dose, 15 ml per kg of body weight (called a loading dose), is initially given for a two-hour period. It is followed by a maintenance dose, 1.5 ml per kg of body weight per hour. Shortly after the initiation of the medication, the woman becomes intoxicated, experiencing nausea, vomiting, headache, restlessness, and sometimes respiratory depression. Her physical safety becomes a prime concern for the hospital staff. She is kept in bed with the side rails up and padded. She is not left alone. She is kept NPO, since aspiration of vomitus is likely. Her respiratory status needs to be evaluated carefully. The fetal heart rate needs to be monitored frequently as ethyl alcohol readily crosses the placenta. Usually 24 hours after discontinuation of the medication, all ill effects of the medication have ceased.

Magnesium sulfate is another tocolytic agent that is occasionally used. Along with stopping uterine contractions, it has the potential for depressing the CNS and cardiac, skeletal, and smooth muscles. Careful assessment needs to be made of initial signs and symptoms of toxicity; they are severe thirst, hot-all-over feeling, and decreased patellar reflex.

Appropriate Nursing Measures
When Premature Delivery is Imminent

The medical staff does not always come to the conclusion that a premature labor should or can be arrested. Often an attempt to stop premature labor is unsuccessful. Therefore, it is always important that the nurse working in the labor and delivery area be aware of her responsibilities if a preterm infant should be born.

This is a critical time for the hospital staff and the fetus and also for the expectant parents, who deserve much emotional support. They need to be informed of all changes in status and all procedures being done. At times emergency measures will be necessary, and only brief statements can be given. Further explanation should be given as soon as time permits. The pediatrician and nursery should be notified of the imminent delivery and resuscitation equipment should be assembled. These are precautionary measures that parents usually find comforting. It is further proof that all that can be done will be done for their baby. The nurse should be aware that a small infant may not require complete dilatation of the cervix. The mother should be discouraged from bearing down, since this might cause damage to the soft tissues of the fetal head (if the vertex is the presenting part). Only those medications that are absolutely necessary for the mother should be administered, because most agents cross the placenta to the baby. Parents are usually more accepting of this approach if they are told the reason for it. General anesthesia is not used; a local anesthetic is preferred. A rather large episiotomy is usually performed.

Once birth has occurred, only procedures that are absolutely necessary should be done to the newborn, since injury and infection are easily introduced. Respirations should be established and the baby should be moved to a source of warmth, humidity, and oxygen. The ideal position for the baby is on his back (supine) with the shoulders elevated so that the abdomen is lower than the thorax and the airway is clear; a folded towel or diaper placed under the shoulders and back helps to expand the thoracic cavity. After briefly sharing the baby with his parents, he is usually transferred to a special care nursery.

Review Question

List 5 measures the nurse should take when anticipating the delivery of a preterm infant.

a. _____

b. _____

c. _____

d. _____

e. _____

Answer

Anticipatory care that should be provided for the preterm infant in the labor and delivery area includes:

Notify the pediatrician and nursery.

Assemble resuscitation equipment.

Avoid all medications for the mother.

Anticipate delivery without complete dilatation.

Discourage mother from bearing down.

Perform only those procedures necessary—establish respiration, provide warmth, humidity, and oxygen.

Position baby to facilitate respirations.

Transfer baby to special care nursery if necessary, after the parents have seen the baby.

Variations in Physical Features of the Preterm Infant

The preterm infant is not only at risk for physical survival but also for acceptance by his parents as a human being identified as theirs and worthy of their love. They need to be allowed to see and touch their baby as soon as and as long as conditions permit. These first few minutes (and hours) of close contact with their baby may be crucial for optimal development later in life. Unless the parents come in contact with their newborn, they are justified in believing he will not survive.

The preterm baby has many characteristics that are different from those seen in the term infant. Many of these characteristics are not usually noticed by the mother (and father), but some of them might create anxiety. The nurse should know the normal signs of the preterm infant and should inform the mother of those that seem appropriate. The cardinal signs of the preterm infant are:

1. General appearance: The preterm infant lies flat in a frog-legged position with shoulders, elbows, and knees all touching the mattress. The head is turned to one side. He is inactive with few spontaneous movements.

2. Skin: This is very transparent, shiny, and red owing to superficial blood vessels. Vernix caseosa begins to form at 5 months and increases in amount until 36 weeks when it begins to slough off.

3. Lanugo: At 20 weeks lanugo first appears on the face and shoulders; it vanishes on the face around 28 weeks and small amounts are on the shoulders through 32 to 37½ weeks.

4. Plantar creases: These begin to form on the anterior part of the soles by 34 weeks; there are increasingly more creases the closer he is to term.

5. Breasts: Breast tissue, nipples, and areolae begin to form at 34 weeks; they become 1 cm and raised by term.

6. Ears: They are pliable with little cartilage; when they are manipulated they do not return to their original position.

7. Genitalia: The male has a small penis; the scrotal sac appears undergrown with little pigmentation and few rugal folds, and testes are undescended or in the canal. The female has gaping vulva because of poorly developed labia majora; the labia minora and clitoris are prominent and thick, and viscid mucoid discharge is lacking or very scanty; there is no bloody discharge.

Except for posture, no mention has been made of the preterm's neurologic reflexes. Please refer to Ballard or Dubowitz for those (see Bibliography).

Review Question

Give one normal characteristic for the preterm infant for each of the following:

General appearance: _____

_____

Skin: _____

_____

Lanugo: _____

_____

Plantar creases: _____

_____

Breasts: _____

Ears: _____

Genitalia: _____

Answer

See list in paragraph on page 161.

Psychologic Tasks for Mothers of Preterm Infants

The nurse must realize the crisis potential that premature labor and possible delivery of a preterm infant has for a mother. Throughout this chapter it has been stressed that the infant has many handicaps. Most mothers are aware of some of them and this naturally creates anxiety. At the time of the birth of a preterm infant, the mother and father are faced with working through four psychologic tasks. One, the smaller and more immature the infant, the greater the possibility of death—much more so than with the term infant; even if the infant survives, a period of *grieving normally occurs*. Two, the mother must also admit to the fact that she has not carried this baby the normal length of time; this is likely to create *guilt feelings*, which she must *acknowledge*. Three, assuming that the baby survives, the mother needs to *begin to relate to her baby*—to see it, touch it, care for it. Four, she needs to *gain a realistic understanding* of how her baby differs in its *needs and approaches* from that of a term infant.

Review Question

What are the four psychologic tasks that a mother of a preterm infant must work through?

a. _____
b. _____
c. _____
d. _____

Answer

The mother of a preterm infant must:
a. prepare for possible loss of the infant.

b.   acknowledge failure to deliver a normal full-term infant.
c.   initiate a process of relating to the baby.
d.   understand the special needs of a preterm infant.

How a Nurse can Facilitate Parental-Infant Attachment

The nurse plays a significant role in assisting the parents to accept their new baby. A trusting relationship between the parents and nurse is necessary first. The nurse should accept that both, but especially the mother, may have negative feelings about the premature birth experience. The nurse should encourage them to express these feelings freely and, when necessary, encourage them to seek help with these feelings. The nurse should communicate the infant's progress to the parents, make it possible for them to frequently see and touch their infant, and allow them to care for the infant when possible. When they do something to comfort the baby, they should be praised; positive reinforcement will encourage further parental-infant interaction. They may wonder why the baby startles in such an exaggerated fashion and why he doesn't grasp on to a parent's finger; they need to be assured that these are normal responses of an immature infant. It is a healthy response for parents to ask many questions about their baby; these questions warrant answers that the parents can comprehend. The baby who appears as attractive as possible and who is treated with warmth by the nurses will be more acceptable to the parents. Even though it will require a longer period of time for these parents to identify with and claim their baby, if they can gain confidence in their ability to care for their baby while in the hospital, the parental-infant relationship will be a much more satisfactory one at home.

Review Question

Identify four ways a nurse can promote parental-infant attachment following a premature birth:

a. _____
b. _____
c. _____
d. _____

Answer

A nurse can promote parental-infant attachment in the following ways:
Establish a trusting relationship with the parents.
Accept and work through their negative feelings about the premature birth.

Keep the parents informed about the status of their infant.

Allow them to be with their infant when possible.

Encourage their positive interactions with the baby.

Allow them to ask questions and provide them with answers.

Allow them to gain confidence in caring for their baby.

Death of a Premature Infant

Before concluding this section on preterm labor, at least brief consideration needs to be given to the premature infant who dies, since this is a
possible outcome. Parents need to know about the death of their infant
as soon as possible. At first disbelief will be evident. They should be
encouraged to see their baby, since an unseen baby is imagined to be far
worse than he actually is. Many parents find it helpful to touch or hold
their baby, to take a picture of him, and to give him a name to refer to
him by. These measures help to make the situation real to them. They
will experience distress, irritability, and feelings of guilt and anger. A
funeral service provides an opportunity for them to begin to work through
the grieving process. Preoccupation with thoughts about their baby will
continue for several weeks. During this time the couple needs to support
each other, to talk about the death with each other, and to talk occasionally to one or two professional people—physician, nurse, social worker,
or clergy. Resumption of normal activities should gradually occur. Although
no person or object will ever replace the child they have lost, by 6 to 8
months the couple normally has worked through the grieving process.

POST-TERM LABOR

Effects of Post-term Labor on Mother and Infant

Pregnancy that goes beyond 42 weeks is termed post-dates, prolonged
gestation, or *post-term*. It takes its toll on both mother (and father) and
fetus, as does premature labor.

By 42 weeks the mother has been ready to have her baby for weeks.
She is fatigued and frustrated. The repeated question "Haven't you had
your baby yet?" doesn't help. She begins to lose self-confidence and
becomes critical of her own abilities. Around week 42 her doctor usually
recommends a series of tests to determine the fetal status and to verify
that she is post-term. A previously well-functioning placenta could now
begin to show signs of insufficiency in meeting the needs of the fetus. As
the mother realizes this she begins to fear for the well-being of her baby.

At what post-term age the fetus is compromised is not predictable. Some continue to grow without degeneration in their biologic functioning; some become so large that vaginal delivery becomes difficult. Those who stop growing and lose weight are called *postmature* or *dysmature*.

The post-term infant normally has the following readily identifiable characteristics:

1. General appearance: arms and legs fully flexed; large.
2. Skin: thick, pink, parchmentlike owing to the lack of vernix; may be peeling.
3. Lanugo: little if any.
4. Plantar creases: deep indentations over more than one third of anterior sole.
5. Breasts: tissue, nipples, areolae well-developed.
6. Ears: well-defined, firm pinna.
7. Genitalia: pigmented. Male: numerous rugae, 1 or 2 testes descended. Female: labia majora covering minora and clitoris, bloody discharge possible.

(Note that a comparable list of characteristics is given for the premature infant earlier in this chapter.) The post-term infant may also have signs of *postmature syndrome* (which are found in other dysmature situations, for example, severe pre-eclampsia). Signs of postmaturity include:

a. He is thin and scrawny, with loose fitting skin owing to decreased placental perfusion and use of his own glucose stores.

b. His skin, nails, and cord are often stained with meconium, passed during episodes of anoxia in utero.

c. He appears wide-eyed and alert but worried, which are symptomatic of chronic intrauterine hypoxia.

Review Questions

1. At what time is a fetus classified as post-term? _____
2. What psychologic effects might a prolonged gestation have on a mother?
   a. _____
   b. _____
   c. _____
3. In addition to post-term characteristics, a postmature infant has the following characteristics:
   a. Owing to use of his own glucose stores, he appears _____
      _____
   b. His _____ are often meconium stained.
   c. Chronic intrauterine hypoxia causes him to look _____
      _____

Answers

1.	*Greater than 42 weeks gestation* is classified as post-term.
2.	The psychologic effects of prolonged gestation include: a. fatigue and frustration b. loss of self-confidence; self-doubt c. fear about the well-being of the fetus.
3.	a.	Owing to use of his own glucose stores, the postmature infant appears *thin and scrawny, with loose fitting skin.*
	b.	His *skin, nails, and cord* are often meconium stained.
	c.	Chronic intrauterine hypoxia causes him to look *wide-eyed* and *alert but worried.*

Assessment for Postmaturity

Many of the procedures done to determine the gestational age of the preterm fetus apply here also. The EDC, time of quickening and hearing of the first fetal heart rate, fundal height, BPD via U/S, and amniotic fluid analysis are used to assess the gestational age or fetal growth. Other observations are made to *assess placental function and fetal well-being.* They include urinary estriol excretion, fetal activity tests, oxytocin challenge test, amnioscopy, HPL, and fetal scalp pH.

A common procedure is the collection of *24-hour URINES FOR ESTRIOL EXCRETION.* Because each individual varies in her excretion of estriol in *each* voiding and in *each* 24-hour period, *more than one* 24-hour collection is needed to determine the estriol level. It continues to rise in a healthy pregnancy. A normal level at 34 weeks is greater than 12 mg. The significance of a dropping level is that a source of its production (for example, fetal adrenal and pituitary glands, fetal liver, or placenta) is not functioning properly. Between 4 to 12 mg, a fetus is in jeopardy. Below 4 mg, fetal death is imminent. In order to verify that the entire 24-hour specimen has been obtained, the creatinine level may also be assessed. It is the nurse's role to provide the woman with a container(s) suitable for collection, a refrigeration source (if the lab requires such), and clear instructions about how to collect every voiding in that 24-hour period. The woman should be told that more than one 24-hour collection is routinely necessary. (A few laboratories are capable of testing plasma estriol.)

FETAL ACTIVITY and its effect on the fetal heart rate are indicators of fetal well-being and reserve. A woman may be asked to keep track of her fetal activity. Normally there are three movements within an hour, with a lower limit of 10 in a 12-hour period. Less activity than this warrants further testing.

NONSTRESS TEST (NST), FETAL ACTIVITY ACCELERATION DETERMINATIONS (FAD), OR FETAL ACTIVITY TEST (FAT). This test can be done in an outpatient setting. It is noninvasive and nonhormonal, with no potential side effects. Using an external electronic monitor (described in Chapter 2) the fetal heart rate (FHR) and fetal activity are recorded. In some cases the mother is told to press a button on the fetal monitor at the time she feels fetal movement in order to record the movement on the monitor's graph. Monitoring may need to be continued beyond 20 or 30 minutes, since the lack of activity for that time may be due to the quiet fetal sleep state. Normally the baseline for the FHR varies 5 to 15 BPM, and the rate ranges between 120 and 160. The results of NST are as follows:

a. A healthy fetus experiences an FHR acceleration with fetal movement (a *negative or reactive result*); two or more accelerations of 15 BPM, lasting 15 seconds per 10-minute period are required. A repetition of this test can safely be delayed for one week.

b. Little or no FHR acceleration despite tactile stimulation of the maternal abdomen results in a *positive or nonreactive result*. A fetus with a positive test result is a candidate for OCT.

c. Questionable acceleration or weak, infrequent movements give an *inadequate or suspicious result,* and the test should be repeated in 24 to 48 hours.

OXYTOCIN CHALLENGE TEST. (See Chapter 2 for nursing interventions.) Weekly or semiweekly OCTs are done in the hospital to determine the ability of the post-term fetus to tolerate the stress of uterine contractions. Contraindications to OCT include a history of classic cesarean delivery, placenta previa, and threatening premature labor. An external electronic monitor is applied, and IV oxytocin is given until 3 contractions occur in a 10-minute period. The FHR is assessed in relation to the uterine contractions. Since poor placental perfusion due to an aging placenta is common in the post-term pregnancy, uterine contractions may cause late FHR decelerations (evidence of uteroplacental insufficiency).

The results of OCT are as follows:

a. Consistent late deceleration with most contractions is a *positive test.* Termination of the pregnancy without labor may be necessary.

b. In the presence of inconsistent decelerations it is a *suspicious test.* The OCT should be repeated in 24 hours.

c. Three contractions in 20 minutes without late decelerations is a *negative test.* The test need not be repeated for a week.

AMNIOSCOPY. Viewing of amniotic fluid through the intact amniotic sac is done by inserting a conelike instrument through the cervix vaginally. The procedure is uncomfortable but not painful. The purpose is to detect meconium staining (fetal anoxia) without directly invading the amniotic sac.

HUMAN PLACENTAL LACTOGEN. HPL is a hormone normally produced in progressively larger amounts during pregnancy. Low amounts of HPL have been reported in the blood of mothers with postmature syndrome but further study needs to be done before this hormone can be relied on as a predictor of fetal jeopardy.

FETAL SCALP pH. See Chapter 2 for explanation.

Review Question

Briefly summarize the information you would give to a woman before each of the following tests.
a.   24-hour urine for estriol:
    1.   purpose: _____
    2.   procedure: _____
    _____
    _____

    3.   frequency: _____
    _____

b.   NST:
    1.   purpose: _____
    2.   procedure: _____
    _____
    _____

    3.   frequency: _____
    _____

c.   OCT:
    1.   purpose: _____
    2.   procedure: _____
    _____
    _____

    3.   frequency: _____
    _____

Answer

a.   24-hour urine for estriol:
    1.   purpose: to assess placental functioning

2. procedure: collect all urine passed during a 24-hour period, store it in a designated container(s), refrigerate if required.
3. frequency: routinely at least two 24-hour collections are necessary for comparison
b. Nonstress test:
1. purpose: to assess fetal well-being—the response of the FHR to fetal activity
2. procedure: an external electronic monitor is placed on the abdomen and the FHR and fetal activity recorded; time involved is usually more than 30 minutes
3. frequency: the frequency of repeated tests is dependent on the test results
c. Oxytocin Challenge Test:
1. purpose: to assess fetal well-being—the response of the FHR to uterine contractions stimulated by IV oxytocin
2. procedure: with external electronic monitor in place, IV oxytocin is administered until the effect of uterine contractions on the FHR can be determined. Time involved is usually dependent on the time it takes for the uterus to contract 3 times in 10 minutes
3. frequency: the frequency of the test is dependent on the test results but even good results warrant weekly or semiweekly tests in the post-term pregnancy

Nursing Measures during Post-term Labor

Post-term labor may occur spontaneously or with the aid of stimulants (refer to Chapter 5). Although the mother is undoubtedly relieved that the pregnancy finally is ending, the fetus is about to undergo his most stressful time. Normally, uterine contractions temporarily decrease the amount of oxygenation the fetus receives. If there is any placental insufficiency, which there often is in the post-term pregnancy, the fetus is most frequently compromised during uterine contractions. Careful monitoring of the FHR with a continuous electronic monitor is necessary. Intolerance of uterine contractions is evidenced by persistent late decelerations and decreased baseline variability (refer to Chapter 2) and warrants medical intervention. The nurse should encourage the mother to sit in a semi-Fowler position or to lie on her side to facilitate fetal oxygenation. Oxytocin stimulation, if used, should be regulated to produce contractions of less than 90 seconds duration with a minimum of 60 seconds relaxation between contractions. Intravenous fluids should be administered. Helping the woman to decrease her pain perception is very important, since all medications should be avoided if possible. In the presence of fetal distress, oxygen should be administered to the mother via face mask or nasal cannula. If delivery has not occurred after 12 to 18 hours of good labor, a cesarean delivery is often performed in order to decrease fetal morbidity and mortality.

Review Question

When preparing a mother for her post-term labor what 5 (or more) items would you share with her in expectation of the care she would receive?

a. _____

b. _____

c. _____

d. _____

e. _____

Answer

Items a nurse should share with a woman anticipating a post-term labor are:

a. If labor does not start on its own, it will be stimulated, probably by IV oxytocin.

b. Continuous electronic monitoring will be done.

c. She will be discouraged from lying on her back but encouraged to sit up or lie on her side.

d. IV fluids will be given.

e. Medication will be avoided if possible.

f. If the fetus shows the need for it, oxygen will be given.

g. If necessary a cesarean delivery may be performed.

Immediate Care of the Post-term Infant

In addition to routine newborn care (that is, establishing a patent airway, drying skin, providing warmth, identifying mother and baby, instilling eye prophylaxis), there are special needs that must be met for the post-term infant. The nurse is responsible for notifying the pediatrician and anesthetist when this delivery is imminent, since tracheal suctioning should be done immediately following birth and oxygenation may be administered if bradycardia is present. Suctioning is necessary since aspiration of meconium-stained amniotic fluid is likely to have occurred in utero or at the time of birth. Since the amount of amniotic fluid decreases following 38 weeks, the fluid is often thick and pea-soup—like. If aspirated it would clog the air passages and irritate the lungs. Pneumonitis and possibly pneumothorax could result.

The health team usually checks the newborn for hypoglycemia by means of a Dextrostix. A reading of less than 45 indicates a low blood sugar level, which requires immediate administration of oral or IV glucose solution. Frequent feedings may be necessary. The post-term infant usually has little subcutaneous fat and a large body surface, therefore he is subject to cold stress. Special care must be taken to prevent heat loss and to provide heat to this infant. With these measures, although the post-term infant was at risk while in labor, he often functions well in the nursery.

Review Questions

1. Identify 4 physiologic handicaps that the post-term infant is likely to have that warrant nursing interventions:

   a. _____

   b. _____

   c. _____

   d. _____

2. What nursing actions are necessary for the infant who shows signs of the above physiologic conditions?

   a. _____

   b. _____

   c. _____

   d. _____

Answers

1. Physiologic handicaps that a post-term infant is likely to have that warrant interventions are a. clogged air passages and irritated lungs due to meconium aspiration; b. bradycardia; c. hypoglycemia; and d. cold stress.

2. The nursing actions necessary for the infant who shows signs of the above physiologic conditions include:

   a. provide for pediatrician and anesthetist to be present at delivery so that tracheal suctioning can be immediately performed.

   b. give oxygen as necessary.

   c. check for low blood sugar with Dextrostix. Seek order, if not standing order, for oral or IV glucose solution if results are less than 45.

   d. provide warmth and prevent heat loss.

Bibliography

Affonso, DD and Harris, TR: *Post-term pregnancy: Implications for mother and infant, challenge for the nurse.* J Obstet Gynecol Neonatal Nurs 9:139, 1980.

Ballard, JL, Novak, KK and Driver, M: *A simplified score for assessment of fetal maturation of newly born infants.* J Pediatr 95(5):769, 1979.

Billis, BJ: *Nursing considerations: Administering labor-suppressing medications.* Am J Maternal Child Nurs 5:252, 1980.

Christensen, AA: *Coping with the crisis of a premature birth—One couple's story.* Am J Maternal Child Nurs 2:33, 1977.

Chung, HJ: *Arresting premature labor.* Am J Nurs 76:810, 1976.

Cranley, MS: *Antepartal fetal monitoring.* Am J Nurs 78:2098, 1978.

Diamond, F: *High-risk pregnancy screening techniques: A nursing overview.* J Obstet Gynecol Neonatal Nurs 7:15, 1978.

Dubowitz, LM, Dubowitz, V, and Goldberg, C: *Clinical assessment of gestational age.* J Pediatr 77:1, 1970.

Gabbe, SG: *Assessment of fetal size and growth.* In McNall, LK (ed): *Contemporary Obstetric and Gynecologic Nursing.* CV Mosby, St. Louis, 1980.

Haesslein, HC: *Premature labor.* In Niswander, KR (ed): *Manual of Obstetrics.* Little, Brown & Co, Boston, 1979.

Hallman, M and Teramo, K: *Amniotic fluid phospholipid profile as a predictor of fetal maturity in diabetic pregnancies.* Obstet Gynecol 54(6):703, 1979.

Haney, AF: *Fetal measurements.* Ob/Gyn, Pediatrics & Perinatal Care. 2(9):22, 1978.

Hawkins-Walsh, E: *Diminishing anxiety in parents of sick newborns.* Am J Maternal Child Nurs 5(1):30, 1980.

Hayes, AH, et al (eds): *Ritodrine update.* FDA Drug Bulletin 12(1):4, 1982.

Hildebrand, WL and Schreiner, RL: *Helping parents cope with perinatal death.* Am Fam Physician 22(5):121, 1980.

Hogan, K and Tchang, D: *The role of the nurse during amniocentesis.* J Obstet Gynecol Nurs 7(5):24, 1978.

Hutzel Hospital (Detroit, Michigan) *Labor/delivery nursing protocol: Ritodrine.*

Jensen, MD, Benson, RC, and Bobak, IM: *Maternity Care,* ed 2. CV Mosby, St. Louis, 1981.

Johnson, SH: *High-Risk Parenting.* JB Lippincott, Philadelphia, 1979.

Kaplan, D and Mason, E: *Maternal reactions to premature birth viewed as an acute emotional disorder.* In Parad, HJ (ed): *Crisis Intervention.* Family Service Association of America, New York, 1965.

Kohn, CL, Nelson, A, and Weiner, S: *Gravidas' response to realtime ultrasound fetal image.* J Obstet Gynecol Nurs 9(2):77, 1980.

Kopf, R: *Nonstress test.* Am J Nurs 78:2115, 1978.

Merkatz, IR, Peter, JB, and Barden, TP: *Ritodrine hydrochloride: A betamimetic agent for the use in preterm labor. II. Evidence of efficacy.* Obstet Gynecol 56(1):7, 1980.

MINER, H: *Problems and prognosis for the small-for-gestational age and the premature infant.* Am J Maternal Child Nurs 3(4):221, 1978.

NIEBYL, JR AND JOHNSON, JW: *Inhibition of preterm labor.* Clin Obstet Gynecol 23(1):115, 1980.

OXORN, H: *Oxorn-Foote: Human Labor and Birth,* ed 4. Appleton-Century-Crofts, New York, 1980.

Physicians' Desk Reference, ed 35. Medical Economics Co, Oradell, NJ, 1981.

RAUSCH, PB: *Effects of tactile and kinesthetics stimulation on premature infants.* J Obstet Gynecol Nurs 10(1):34, 1981.

RAYBURN, W AND CHANG, F: *Management of the uncomplicated postdate pregnancy.* J Reprod Med 26(2):93, 1981.

ROTHFEDER, B AND BURDIN, C: *The high-risk infant and family.* In SCIPIEN, GM, ET AL: *Comprehensive Pediatric Nursing.* McGraw-Hill, New York, 1979.

SULLIVAN, R, FOSTER, J, AND SCHREINER, R: *Determining a newborn's gestational age.* Am J Maternal Child Nurs 4(1):38, 1979.

TUCKER, SM: *Fetal Monitoring and Fetal Assessment in High-Risk Pregnancy.* CV Mosby, St. Louis, 1978.

WHEELER, LA AND DUXBURY, ML: *Module 3: Fetal Assessment.* National Foundation/March of Dimes, New York, 1979.

ZIEGEL, EE AND CRANLEY, MS: *Obstetric Nursing,* ed 7. Macmillan, New York, 1978.

POST-TEST

1. On the time line below, *circle* the numerals (representing weeks gestation) that pertain to preterm and post-term and *label* them.

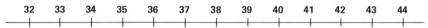

| 32 | 33 | 34 | 35 | 36 | 37 | 38 | 39 | 40 | 41 | 42 | 43 | 44 |

2. In the chart below, list the psychologic effects a nonterm labor might have on a woman:

PREMATURE	POST-TERM
a. _____	a. _____
b. _____	b. _____
c. _____	c. _____

3. Specify which physiologic handicaps tend to occur in the preterm infant and which in the post-term/postmature infant. Indicate PRE and POST in the blanks.

   a. _____ difficult respirations due to surfactant level in lungs

   b. _____ loose fitting skin, deprived looking

   c. _____ parchmentlike, peeling skin

d. _____ weak suck

e. _____ hemorrhage

f. _____ meconium staining

g. _____ poor resistance to infection

4. Explain 3 methods nurses use to determine the gestational age of a fetus and state the normal findings:

   EXAMPLE: To determine the EDC (using Naegele's rule) subtract 3 months and add 7 days and one year to date of onset of LMP. LMP = 7/13/83; EDC = 4/20/84.

   a._____

   _____

   _____

   b._____

   _____

   _____

   c. _____

   _____

   _____

5. List the following physical features in a preterm infant and a post-mature infant.

	PRETERM	POSTMATURE
a. position		
b. vernix		
c. plantar creases		
d. pinna of ears		
e. majora/minora		

6. Explain why the nurse assesses the fetal heart rate in the following procedures:

   a. Amniocentesis: _____

   _____

   _____

   b. Nonstress Test: _____

   _____

   _____

   c. Oxytocin Challenge Test: _____

   _____

   _____

7. Match the drugs in Column I with the appropriate statement in Column II

I	II
a. Betamethasone	_____ May cause pulmonary
b. Ethyl alcohol	edema when given with
c. Ritodrine	other drugs

d. Terbutaline   _____ Has few side effects other
e. Vasodilan   than maternal tachycardia
                                 _____ Physical safety is a prime
                                         concern
                                 _____ Contractions become
                                         stronger, less frequent

8. True-False. Circle the correct answer.
   When premature delivery is imminent, the nurse should:
   a. T   F   Inform the mother of the handicaps her baby will
                 have.
   b. T   F   Provide the mother with enough medication so that
                 she is comfortable both mentally and physically.
   c. T   F   Inform the mother that the baby will be taken to
                 the nursery where he can be given a warm environ-
                 ment and can be closely watched.
   d. T   F   Let the mother know that both the nursery and the
                 pediatrician have been informed that her baby is on
                 his way.
   e. T   F   The mother should be discouraged from bearing
                 down even following complete dilatation.
9. A premature infant's mother must work through the psychologic
   tasks listed below. At the same time a maternal-infant bond needs
   to be promoted. Indicate how a nurse can promote a favorable bond,
   considering the tasks the mother must go through.

PSYCHOLOGIC TASKS	NURSING INTERVENTION
a. feel grief and guilt	a.
b. initiate relationship with baby	b.
c. understand baby's needs	c.

10. Explain why the following measures are carried out during a post-term labor/delivery:
    a. Continuous electronic monitoring:

    _____

    _____

    _____

    b. Tracheal suctioning of newborn:

    _____

    _____

    _____

    c. Dextrostix test:

    _____

    _____

    _____

Answers

1.

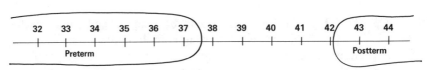

2. The psychologic effects a nonterm labor might have on a woman:

PREMATURE	POSTMATURE
a. has not completed nesting	a. fatigued, frustrated
b. has not let go of imcompatible practices	b. lacking self-confidence
c. not ready to separate from fetus	c. fearful of fetal well-being
d. fears losing or hurting baby	

3. Physiologic handicaps that tend to occur in PREterm and POSTterm:
    a. PRE   difficult respirations due to surfactant levels
    b. POST   loose fitting skin, deprived looking
    c. POST   parchmentlike, peeling skin
    d. PRE   weak suck
    e. PRE   hemorrhage
    f. POST   meconium staining
    g. PRE   poor resistance to infection

4. Signs by which nurses can determine gestational age and the normal time of occurrence for signs:
    a. Ask the mother when she first felt fetal movement (quickening). Normally it occurs at 16 to 18 weeks.

b. Auscultate the *fetal heart rate.* Expect to first hear it with a Doppler device at 10 to 12 weeks, and for the first time with a fetoscope at 18 to 20 weeks.

c. Measure the *fundal height* from the upper border of the symphysis pubis to the top of the fundus. At 16 weeks, it is midway between pubis and umbilicus; at 20 weeks, at umbilicus; at 24 weeks, just above umbilicus.

		PRETERM	POST-TERM
a.	position	frog-legged/extended	fully flexed
b.	vernix	maximum at 36 weeks	lacking
c.	plantar creases	some on anterior sole	deep; over more than 1/3 of anterior sole
d.	pinna or ears	pliable/floppy	firm
e.	majora/minora	minora prominent	majora covering minora

6. Why fetal heart rate assessment is done:
   a. Amniocentesis: Injury of the fetus, cord, or placenta may occur due to penetration with the needle used to withdraw the amniotic fluid.
   b. Nonstress Test: NST specifically looks for accelerations in FHR upon fetal movement. A healthy fetus experiences an FHR acceleration with each fetal movement. Lack of accelerations warrants further assessment.
   c. Oxytocin Challenge Test: OCT specifically looks for the FHR response to uterine contractions. It is abnormal for the fetus to experience late decelerations, which is fairly common in the post-term fetus.

7. a. Betamethasone: May stimulate pulmonary edema in mother
   b. Ethyl alcohol: Physical safety is a prime concern
   c. Ritodrine: Has few side effects other than maternal tachycardia
   d. Terbutaline: (no correct response)
   e. Vasodilan: Contractions become stronger and less frequent.

8. a. F; b. F; c. T; d. T; e. T.

9.

MATERNAL PSYCHOLOGIC TASKS	NURSING INTERVENTIONS
a. feel grief and guilt	a. accept/work through mother's negative feelings
b. initiate relationship with baby	b. allow mother to be with baby
c. understand baby's needs	c. allow for and answer mother's questions

10. During a post-term labor/delivery, the following measures are done:
    a. Continuous electronic monitoring: Assess for signs of placen-

tal insufficiency (late decelerations in FHR) with contractions.

b.   Tracheal suctioning of newborn: In the presence of meconium-stained amniotic fluid, aspiration would cause respiratory distress.

c.   Dextrostix test: Hypoglycemia is common in post-term infants and requires early diagnosis and treatment (early, frequent glucose feedings).

CHAPTER 7

PAIN RELIEF VIA DRUGS DURING LABOR AND DELIVERY

Carolyn Pedigo DeLoach

This chapter has been prepared to help you understand the importance of the proper use of drugs for relief of pain, tension, and anxiety during labor and delivery. The concept of pain is included to help you assess the presence and degree of pain experienced by a patient in labor in order to determine the need for drug intervention. Partial or full relief of pain may be achieved with drugs at various times. Safety is the main focus whenever drugs are administered during labor and delivery. The degree of safety is determined by assessing the direct effects of drugs upon the mother and how these may indirectly affect the fetus or newborn. The major focus of this chapter is pain relief through drugs; decreased perception of pain through hypnosis and childbirth classes is discussed in Chapter 8.

A suggested prerequisite to this chapter is a basic understanding of the normal anatomy and physiology of the reproductive system in relation to the labor and delivery process. A pharmacology book should be consulted for additional information about the drugs mentioned throughout this chapter.

OBJECTIVES

Upon completion of this chapter, the reader will be able to:

1. Explain the subjective aspects of pain and identify four current theories regarding the cause of pain in labor.

continued on next page

2. Define analgesia and anesthesia as they are used in obstetrics.
3. List three detrimental side effects of pain.
4. Identify three considerations that may influence the decision of whether or not to use drugs in labor. List three direct effects of drugs that may be considered undesirable for the mother, and three indirect effects on the fetus or newborn, and the appropriate nursing interventions.
5. Discuss five supportive nursing measures that may be used in conjunction with drugs to decrease pain perception.
6. Discuss the action and side effects of analgesics, sedative-hypnotics, amnesics, and tranquilizers commonly used in labor (specifically: Demerol, barbiturates, scopolamine, Phenergan, Vistaril, and Sparine).
7. Differentiate between the different types of anesthesia used during labor and delivery (paracervical, spinal, saddle, caudal, epidural, and pudendal blocks, local perineal infiltration, inhalation and intravenous anesthesia).
8. Describe methods of assessing the effectiveness of analgesia and anesthesia.
9. Describe emergency nursing measures that may be carried out as a result of complications following the administration of anesthesia.

DRUGS COMMONLY USED DURING LABOR

Subjective Aspects of Pain and Theories on the Cause of Pain

Labor and delivery can be a fascinating and exciting time for the expectant family. It is the culmination of pregnancy and also the beginning of the long-awaited birth of the child. The term labor means work, and yet, that term has many other associations. Unfortunately, the major association in our society is that of *pain*.

Pain is a subjective phenomenon. Pain exists when an individual experiences a sensation, interprets the sensation as painful, and exhibits a psychologic and physiologic reaction to the sensation. Perception of pain during labor may be intensified by progressive uterine contractions, fatigue, lack of sleep, anxiety, and fears. Previous experience with pain, personal expectations of pain in labor, and one's own cultural concept of pain will also affect the perception of pain and the individual's response to pain. Physiologic reactions to pain may include increases in blood pressure, heart rate, respirations, perspiration, and pupil diameter and muscle tension (fisted hands, rigidity, grimacing, facial tension) or muscle activity (twisting, turning, pacing). Verbal expressions of pain may include statements about pain, cries for help, and moaning and groaning. Nonverbal expressions of pain may include depression, withdrawal, hostility, and fear.

Owing to the total subjectivity of pain, no *one* cause of pain in labor has been determined. Numerous theories about the causes of pain in labor have been hypothesized. Some are:

1. *Anoxia* of compressed muscle cells of the uterus brought about with each contraction;
2. *Compression* of the nerve ganglia in the cervix and lower uterine segments during contractions;
3. *Stretching* of the cervix during dilatation and effacement;
4. *Stretching* and displacement of the perineum as the fetus descends through the birth canal;
5. *Pressure* on the urethra, bladder, and rectum as the fetus descends; and
6. *Fear* resulting in tension that causes pain and more fear as a spontaneous occurrence.

Review Questions

1. Pain is a subjective phenomenon that exists when an individual:
   a. _____
   b. _____
   c. _____

2. Identify 4 factors that may intensify a woman's perception of pain during labor.
   a. _____
   b. _____
   c. _____
   d. _____

3. Identify 3 physiologic and 3 behavioral indications of pain perception.
   Physiologic: Behavioral (verbal or nonverbal):
   a. _____   a. _____
   b. _____   b. _____
   c. _____   c. _____

4. List four theories of the cause of pain in labor.
   a. _____
   b. _____
   c. _____
   d. _____

Answers

1. Pain exists when an individual: a. experiences a sensation, b. interprets the sensation as painful, and c. exhibits a psychologic and physiologic reaction to the sensation.

2. Factors that may intensify a woman's perception of pain during labor include: a. progressive labor contractions, b. fatigue, c. lack of sleep, d. personal expectations of pain in labor, and e. cultural concept of pain.

3. Indications of pain perception. Physiologic reactions include increased: a. blood pressure, b. heart rate, c. respirations, e. pupil diameter, f. muscle tension, g. muscle activity.
   Behavioral reactions may be verbal or nonverbal including: a. statements about pain, b. cries for help, c. moaning and groaning, d. depression, e. withdrawal, f. hostility, g. fear.

4. Current theories of the cause of pain in labor are:
   a. anoxia of compressed muscle cells of the uterus brought about with each contraction;
   b. compression of the nerve ganglia in the cervix and lower uterine segments during contractions;
   c. stretching of the cervix during dilatation and effacement;
   d. stretching and displacement of the perineum as the fetus descends through the birth canal;
   e. pressure on the urethra, bladder, and rectum as the fetus descends; and
   f. fear resulting in tension that causes pain and more fear as a spontaneous occurrence.

Analgesia and Anesthesia in Obstetrics

Labor and delivery should be a positive family experience. Yet that sounds contradictory in view of the pain that normally accompanies labor and delivery. Therefore, the purpose of analgesia and anesthesia, in obstetrics as well as other areas, is to provide as much relief from pain as possible through pharmaceutical intervention. At the same time it is important that undesirable side effects of drugs on the fetus, the newborn, and the mother be kept to a minimum. All medications received by the woman in labor can cross the placenta and affect the fetus. The selection of analgesia and anesthesia is frequently one of the most important decisions made in the management of the labor patient.

During Stage I of labor, pain impulses (Fig. 7-1) due to uterine contractions and cervical dilatation are transmitted by nerve fibers from

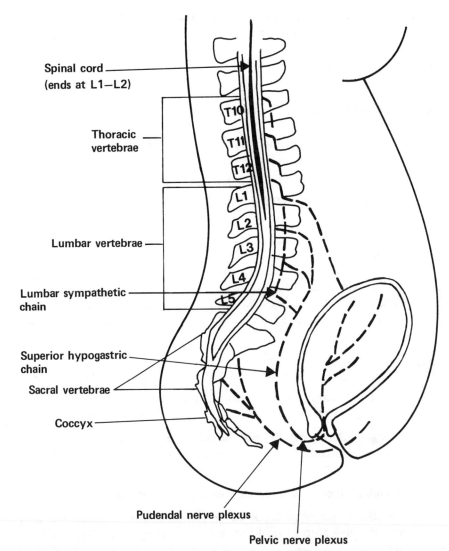

Spinal cord
(ends at L1—L2)

Thoracic
vertebrae

T10

T11

T12

L1

L2

L3

L4

L5

Lumbar vertebrae

Lumbar sympathetic
chain

Superior hypogastric
chain

Sacral vertebrae

Coccyx

Pudendal nerve plexus

Pelvic nerve plexus

Figure 7-1. Uterine impulse (pain) pathway to the spinal canal.

the cervix and uterus to T-10, T-11, and T-12 (thoracic nerves) and L-1 (lumbar nerve). Pain relief during Stage I interferes with pain impulses reaching the spinal canal or provides systemic relief of pain. During Stage II, perineal pain impulses are transmitted by the pudendal nerve to S-2, S-3, and S-4 (sacral nerves).[1] Pain relief for delivery blocks pain at the levels of S-2 through S-4 or provides systemic relief of pain.

What is meant by analgesia and anesthesia? *Analgesia* refers to the absence or decreased awareness of a normal sensation of pain; it is brought about most often by the use of drugs and is usually employed during

Stage I of labor. *Anesthesia* refers to a partial or complete loss of sensation with or without loss of consciousness; it is also brought about most often by the use of drugs and is usually employed toward the end of Stage I and during Stages II and III of labor.

Review Questions

1. Pain relief during Stage I may be accomplished by blocking pain impulses at the spinal levels of _____ .

2. Pain relief during delivery may be achieved by blocking pain impulses from the pudendal nerve at the spinal levels of _____ _____ .

3. Analgesia refers to: _____
    _____
    _____

4. Anesthesia refers to: _____
    _____
    _____

Answers

1. Pain relief during the first stage of labor may be accomplished by blocking pain impulses at the spinal levels of *T-10 through L-1.*

2. Pain relief during delivery may be achieved by blocking pain impulses from the pudendal nerve at the spinal levels of *S-2, S-3, and S-4.*

3. *Analgesia* refers to the absence or decreased awareness of a normal sensation of pain. It is usually employed during Stage I.

4. *Anesthesia* refers to a partial or complete loss of sensation. It is usually employed toward the end of Stage I and during Stages II and III.

Detrimental Side Effects of Pain

Now that you are familiar with the terms analgesia and anesthesia, look at some of the detrimental side effects of experiencing excessive pain so that you have a better understanding of the necessity for pain relief. Pain experienced by the woman in labor can cause:
    1. increased cardiac output (15 to 60 percent),
    2. increased blood pressure and pulse rate,

3. alterations in the function of the uterus, genitourinary tract, and skeletal muscles, leading to spasms of these muscles,
4. nausea and vomiting,
5. possible prolongation of labor, and
6. postpartum emotional reactions such as a delayed development of the normal maternal-infant relationship.

Review Question

List at least three side effects of pain that could be detrimental to the woman in labor:

1. _____
2. _____
3. _____

Answers

Detrimental effects of pain for the woman in labor are:
1. increased cardiac output,
2. increased blood pressure and pulse rate,
3. alterations in the function of the uterus, genitourinary tract, and skeletal muscles.
4. nausea and vomiting,
5. possible prolongation of labor, and
6. postpartum interruption of the development of the maternal-infant relationship.

Considerations That Influence the Decision to Use Drugs

Since excessive pain perception can be detrimental, it is evident that decreasing the sensation of pain is desirable and often necessary. In choosing a method of pain relief, keep in mind the objective of providing as much relief from pain as possible without causing undesirable medication side effects on the mother, fetus, or newborn. The following considerations must be carefully made:
1. Potency of the drug: the drug should be potent enough to relieve pain yet have only minimal side effects on the mother, fetus, or newborn.
2. Possible side effects on the mother, fetus, or newborn: direct effects on the mother cause indirect effects on the fetus or newborn in the following ways:

a. impaired ventilation or arterial hypotension of the mother can cause decreased fetal oxygenation with decreased fetal heart rates,

b. arterial hypertension of the mother can cause abruption of the placenta with fetal anoxia and possible death, and

c. alteration in the forces of labor can cause fetal trauma due to prolonged labor.

3. Stage of labor and progress made:

a. if pain intervention is employed too early (before 4 cm dilatation), it may temporarily interfere with the progress of labor, stopping or slowing down the frequency, intensity, and duration of the contractions,

b. if analgesia is employed late in labor (within 30 to 60 minutes of delivery), it may lead to the delivery of a sedated newborn who may need resuscitative measures. This is usually seen in a newborn with low Apgar scores, and

c. if analgesic intervention is employed in the active labor patient (usually between 4 to 6 cm dilatation) it can decrease or omit the experienced pain so that the labor patient is able to relax and labor may progress at an optimal rate.

Review Questions

1. List three considerations that must be investigated before initiating analgesia or anesthesia to provide pain relief without undesirable side effects:

a. _____

b. _____

c. _____

2. List three possible direct effects on the mother that indirectly cause effects on the fetus or newborn:

a. _____

b. _____

c. _____

Answers

1. Before initiating analgesia or anesthesia to provide pain relief without undesirable side effects, the following considerations must be made:

a. potency of the drug,

b. side effects on the mother and fetus/newborn,

c. stage of labor and progress made.

2. Direct effects on the mother that indirectly cause effects on the fetus or newborn include:
    a. impaired ventilation or arterial hypotension can cause decreased fetal oxygenation causing decreased fetal heart rate,
    b. arterial hypertension can cause placental abruption leading to fetal anoxia and possible death, and
    c. alteration in the forces of labor can cause fetal trauma due to prolonged labor.

Supportive Nursing Measures
Used in Conjunction with Drugs

If labor and delivery are believed to be a painful experience and if drugs can be given to alleviate that pain, then how can the nurse be important in providing pain relief during the labor and delivery experience? *Drugs alone are not the answer.* The nurse can be successful or ineffective depending on her understanding of the physiologic and psychologic aspects involved in this maturational crisis of labor and delivery.

In order to help a patient cope with pain the nurse needs to first determine the patient's perception of the experience. Nursing assessment should include acknowledgment of whether or not pain is present, the patient's description of the characteristics of the pain, and the meaning of the pain experience to the patient. According to McCaffery, "Pain is whatever the experiencing person says it is and exists whenever he says it does."[2] Explore how much the patient knows about pain. How does she feel about the pain experience? Does she want relief from the pain? Does she know what she can do to help reduce the pain? Does she know that drugs can alleviate the pain?

Effective nursing interventions that might be employed as a means of support are:
1. *teaching* or reinforcing relaxation techniques,
2. *encouraging* comfortable and appropriate breathing patterns throughout contractions,
3. *praising* positive efforts made by the couple,
4. *promoting* rest between contractions,
5. *informing* the couple of effective progress throughout labor,
6. *accurately assessing* reactions to pain and need for analgesia, and
7. *assessing* the effectiveness of analgesics used while observing for potential side effects.

Review Question

List 5 measures the nurse can use or suggest in giving support.
1. _____

2. _____
3. _____
4. _____
5. _____

Answers

The nurse might use or suggest the following supportive measures:
1. relaxation techniques,
2. comfortable breathing patterns,
3. praising the couple's positive efforts,
4. rest between contractions,
5. informing couple of progress,
6. assessing need for analgesia, and
7. assessing effectivenes of analgesics used.

The Action and Side Effects of Drugs Commonly Used During Labor

Systemic drugs most commonly used during labor may be classified as: (1) analgesics and narcotic antagonists; (2) sedative-hypnotics; (3) amnesics; and (4) tranquilizers.

ANALGESICS. Analgesics are narcotic or synthetic narcotic (opium based) drugs that are effective in relieving pain 75 to 90 percent of the time. Analgesics also produce sedation, antispasmodic action, euphoria, and decreased anxiety. Side effects of analgesics include nausea and vomiting, respiratory and circulatory depression, delayed gastrointestinal action, and urine retention. Narcotics given 1 to 3 hours prior to delivery may produce neonatal respiratory depression, because the narcotic is synthesized by the fetal liver and activated within the fetal system during that period of time.[3] A good rule of thumb is to *refrain from administering narcotics* after complete dilatation in the primigravida and after 7 to 8 cm dilatation in the multigravida. Analgesics that may be used in labor include morphine sulfate, meperidine hydrochloride (Demerol), pentazocaine (Talwin), oxycodone (Percodan), and codeine.

    The most common synthetic narcotic used during labor is Demerol which is administered IM or IV in dosages of 25 to 100 mg, depending on the route and the woman's body weight. Demerol 50 to 100 mg IM will have an onset of action within 15 minutes and provide analgesia for 1½ to 2 hours. The onset of action when administered IV (usually 50 mg or less) is 3 to 5 minutes lasting 1½ to 2 hours. When administering IV

Demerol, injection during the peak (acme) of a contraction is thought to decrease placental transfer of the drug to the fetus. The oral route is rarely used owing to decreased gastric absorption during labor.

Demerol, if administered at the appropriate time, may promote cervical relaxation producing increased progress of labor. If given too early in labor, it may temporarily disrupt the labor pattern and prolong labor. It is generally recommended that Demerol *not be* administered before 5 to 6 cm dilatation in the primigravida and 3 to 4 cm in the multigravida. This is only a guide. The character and progression of the woman's labor must be carefully evaluated to determine the most appropriate time for administration of Demerol.

Demerol administered during labor may also cause subtle behavioral changes in the newborn during the first 24 hours of life and possibly longer. *These newborns tend to be less alert and generally demonstrate sluggish behavior. They exhibit a decreased response to maternal stimuli such as startling, cuddling, and consoling.*[3,4,5] It may be difficult to help the new mother understand that her baby will become more alert and responsive with time. The new mother has a need to feel adequate in her ability to care for her baby particularly through her ability to feed him. She may feel quite frustrated and sometimes inadequate when he is too sluggish to eat. Supportive nursing intervention is of particular importance at this time.

Stadol (butorphanol tartrate) is a potent nonnarcotic analgesic with narcotic antagonist properties. It is a relatively new drug that is gaining in popularity for use during labor and delivery. The duration of analgesia is 3 to 4 hours and is approximately equal to morphine. The onset of action is 10 minutes with IM administration and very rapid when given IV. The usual single dose is 2 mg; Stadol 1 to 4 mg may be given every 3 to 4 hours. The major side effects are respiratory depression, nausea, and sweating. If respiratory depression occurs, it can be reversed with naloxone.

NARCOTIC ANTAGONISTS. The major side effect of narcotics is respiratory depression. *Narcotic antagonists,* which include nalorphine (Nalline), levallorphan tartrate (Lorfan), and naloxone (Narcan), are administered to reverse the respiratory depression caused by narcotics *only.* If respiratory depression is caused by other factors such as head or cord compression or placental insufficiency, narcotic antagonists will only enhance that depression. Narcotic antagonists may also increase the depression caused by barbiturates, tranquilizers, and sedatives. Narcotic antagonists are administered in one of the following ways to counteract narcotic respiratory depression of the fetus or newborn: (1) IM or IV administration of Nalline 2.5 to 5 mg, Lorfan 0.1 mg, or Narcan 0.4 mg to the mother 5 to 15 minutes prior to delivery; and (2) IM administration or IV administration to the neonate through the umbilical vein immediately after birth of a dilute solution of Nalline 0.05, Lorfan 0.1, or Narcan 0.01 mg per kg of body weight. Hodgkinson et al[6] found that Narcan administered to the mother 15 minutes prior to delivery does reverse the narcotic depression in the neonate at 2 hours of age. However, at 4 and 24 hours of age, these babies displayed almost as much depressed neurobehavior as newborns exposed to Demerol alone. Therefore, they recommend reversing narcotic respiratory and neurobehavioral depression of the neonate by administering Narcan to the newborn immediately after birth.

Review Questions

1. List three actions of analgesics.
   a. _____
   b. _____
   c. _____

2. The major fetal or neonatal side effect of analgesic administration during labor is: _____
   _____

3. Narcotic antagonists used to reverse the major side effect of narcotics are _____, _____, and _____ .

Answers

1. Analgesics used during labor produce a. pain relief, b. sedation, c. antispasmodic action, d. euphoria, and e. decreased anxiety.

2. The major fetal or neonatal side effect of analgesics is *respiratory depression of the mother and fetus/newborn*.

3. *Nalline, Lorfan, and Narcan* are narcotic antagonists used to reverse the respiratory depression caused by narcotics *only*.

SEDATIVE-HYPNOTICS. Sedative-hypnotics are drugs that *do not relieve pain*. They are used during labor to enhance emotional well-being, promote rest and sleep, and potentiate the action of narcotics, thereby decreasing the amount of narcotic needed. Sedative-hypnotic drugs most commonly used are *barbiturates* such as sodium secobarbital (Seconal), sodium pentobarbital (Nembutal), and amobarbital (Amytal). The usual dosage is 100 to 200 mg (o) or 50 to 100 mg IM. Barbiturates cause sedation, relaxation, some hypnosis, and no amnesia; however, recollection may be confused or distorted. They are used in false labor or early labor (1 to 3 cm dilatation) to decrease apprehension, fear, and anxiety, and thereby, decrease the patient's reaction to pain. Barbiturates may produce restlessness when used alone in the presence of moderate to severe pain.

Barbiturates rapidly cross the placenta (in 30 to 60 seconds IV; in 3 to 5 minutes IM) and accumulate in the fetal liver and central nervous system. The following significant neonatal behavioral changes have been identified in newborns whose mothers received barbiturates during labor: *During the first four days of life, these infants exhibit a poor sucking reflex, fewer sucks per minute, lower sucking pressure, and decreased formula intake as compared with infants whose mothers had not received barbiturates during labor.*[7] ˙

AMNESICS. *Scopolamine* is a sedative and tranquilizer with amnesic qualities. The usual dose is 0.2 to 0.6 mg IM or IV. It potentiates the action of narcotics and is used in conjunction with Demerol. Although the anticipated action of scopolamine is sedation and amnesia, undesirable side effects frequently predominate. These side effects include *disorientation, loss of initiative, feelings of helplessness, visual and auditory hallucinations, and marked excitement and delirium.* It is difficult, sometimes impossible, to communicate with a patient who has received scopolamine. Scopolamine also crosses the placenta, rapidly causing fetal depression.

Stop a minute and try to visualize a person exhibiting the above side effects. Now add to your mental picture the normal psychophysical reactions to active labor. Can you imagine the lack of physical and mental control and the loss of all ability to cope once psychologic control barriers are down as a result of scopolamine? And yet, owing to its amnesic qualities, the patient remembers little if any of her behavior during the period of drug action. These patients often express what a fantastic labor they had. They think they were knocked out and slept through the entire process. How mortified they might be if they actually could remember their behavior during that period. There is a fragmented memory or no memory at all of disorientation, loss of initiative, feelings of helplessness, visual and auditory hallucinations, and marked excitement and delirium. Yet one or all may have occurred.

Postpartally, a mother needs to comprehend the reality of labor and delivery by reviewing and ordering the events in her mind. She can then move into the present and begin the maternal-infant bonding process. Scopolamine blocks this assimilation owing to its amnesic qualities and may prolong the comprehension phase which would delay the attachment process.

Review Questions

1. Barbiturates may be used in early labor to decrease:
   a. _____
   b. _____
   c. _____

2. List three behavioral changes observed in the newborn during the first four days of life following barbiturate administration to the mother during labor.
   a. _____
   b. _____
   c. _____

3. Scopolamine is a hypnotic amnesic drug. List four undesirable side effects on the mother.
   a. _____
   b. _____
   c. _____
   d. _____

Answers

1. Barbiturates may be used in early labor to decrease: a. apprehension, b. fear, c. anxiety, and d. the patient's reaction to pain.

2. Newborn behavioral changes associated with barbiturate administration to the mother during labor may include: a. poor sucking reflex, b. fewer sucks per minute, c. lower sucking pressure, and d. decreased formula intake.

3. Scopolamine may produce the following side effects when administered to a woman in labor: a. disorientation, b. loss of initiative, c. feelings of helplessness, d. visual and auditory hallucinations, e. marked excitement and delirium, and f. delayed maternal-infant attachment process.

TRANQUILIZERS. Tranquilizers, also called ataractics, *do not relieve pain.* They may be given alone in early labor (1 to 3 cm dilatation) to decrease apprehension and anxiety, to promote sedation and tranquility, and to relieve nausea. When combined with analgesics, they potentiate the narcotic actions thus reducing the total amount of analgesic needed. They also potentiate the action of sedatives and are used to counteract the hyperactivity caused by scopolamine.

Tranquilizers include promazine (Sparine) 50 mg, promethazine (Phenergan) 25 to 50 mg, hydroxyzine (Vistaril) 25 to 50 mg, and diazepam (Valium) 5 to 10 mg. The major side effect of tranquilizers is maternal hypotension with resulting decreased fetal oxygenation. Phenergan is thought to affect the attention span of the newborn after birth.[8] Intrapartum administration of Valium may cause newborn hypothermia and hypotonia.[9,10]

Review Question

List three actions of tranquilizers.

a. _____

b. _____

c. _____

Answers

Tranquilizers may be given during labor a. to decrease apprehension and anxiety, b. to promote sedation and tranquility, c. to relieve nausea, d. to potentiate action of sedatives and analgesics, and e. to counteract the hyperactivity caused by scopolamine.

In conclusion, sedative-hypnotics, amnesics, and tranquilizers are usually given in early labor to decrease anxiety, promote rest and sleep in the fatigued patient, and potentiate the action of narcotics. It is common for the unprepared primigravida to enter the hospital in early labor, excited, tense, and anxious, with a cervix one cm dilated and 50 percent effaced, and a history of little sleep. This is not the ideal way to approach the hard work of active labor that lies ahead. The use of sedative-hypnotics or tranquilizers at appropriate times in labor will help her to calm down, to sleep, and to gain the needed rest for her forthcoming task. When she awakens, she may have progressed to 3 to 4 cm dilatation with a great deal more cervical effacement, or she may be more calm, and thus better able to cope with the forces of labor.

The following chart shows the drugs most commonly administered and when they are given during labor. The arrows denote the desired length of action of each drug.

PHASE I Latency (1–3 cm)	PHASE II Early Active (4–7 cm)	PHASE III Late Active (8–10 cm)
	Analgesics (narcotics) (Demerol) – – – – – – ⟶	
	Analgesic narcotics + Narcotic antagonists (Demerol + Lorfan, Nalline, or Narcan) – – – – – – ⟶	
Sedative-hypnotic Barbiturates alone (phenobarbital, Sec- onal, Nembutal)⟶		Narcotic antago- nists alone (Lorfan, Nalline or Narcan)
Amnesics alone⟶ (scopolamine)		
	Amnesics with narcotics – – – – (scopolamine + Demerol) ⟶	
Tranquilizers alone – – ⟶ (Sparine, Phener- gan, Vistaril, Valium)		
	Tranquilizers with narcotics – – – – – – ⟶ (Sparine, Phenergan, Vistaril or Valium + Demerol)	

LABOR — STAGE I. Beginning of labor to complete cervical dilatation.

DRUG-INDUCED ANESTHESIA DURING LABOR AND DELIVERY

Anesthesia, a partial or total loss of sensation with or without loss of consciousness, may be *local, regional,* or *general. Local anesthesia* blocks sensory nerve pathways at the organ level, producing anesthesia to the organ only. *Regional anesthesia* blocks sensory nerve pathways along the large sensory nerves from an organ and its surrounding tissues. *General anesthesia* is a progressive depression of the central nervous system, causing loss of sensation in the entire body and loss of consciousness. Most anesthetic procedures are used at the time of delivery, although some are administered during active labor. General anesthesia is not as commonly used in obstetrics as local and regional anesthetics. Local and regional anesthesia are usually achieved by the injection of a drug such as procaine (Novocain), lidocaine (Xylocaine), tetracaine (Pontocaine), mepivacaine (Carbocaine), chloroprocaine (Nesacaine), and bupivacaine (Marcaine).

There is a wide variation in choice of anesthetic agents according to geographic location. However, the two most commonly recommended local anesthetic agents are Marcaine and Nesacaine. It is believed that Marcaine does not cross the placenta as readily as Xylocaine. Nesacaine provides a wide margin of safety, because it is rapidly metabolized in the blood streams of both mother and fetus.[11,12,13] Carbocaine is thought to be poorly metabolized by the neonate.[14,15,16]

A review of the spinal canal anatomy will be beneficial in understanding drug-induced anesthesia discussed later in this chapter (Fig. 7–2).

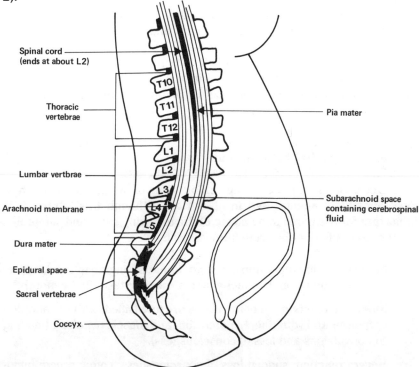

Figure 7-2. Schematic drawing of the spinal canal anatomy.

Nursing care is extremely important before, during, and after the administration of an anesthetic agent because of the possible undesirable side effects that may occur to the mother or fetus. Important nursing measures related to the administration of an anesthetic agent include:

1. *positioning* the patient for the procedure,
2. *providing* emotional support,
3. *monitoring* labor patterns, blood pressure, pulse, and fetal heart rate closely to perceive deviations,
4. *being aware* of and watching for the possible side effects of the anesthetic agent, and
5. *initiating* emergency measures related to maternal hypotension or fetal bradycardia (see Chapter 2).

Emergency Nursing Measures for Complications Following Anesthetic Administration

Maternal hypotension and fetal bradycardia are the most frequently occurring side effects associated with anesthesia. A sudden episode of severe nausea may be the first sign of hypotension. If hypotension occurs, the nurse should:

1. *turn* the mother on her left side to relieve uterine pressure on iliac veins and inferior vena cava and to promote venous return, thereby increasing oxygen supply to the fetus,
2. *administer* oxygen at 5 to 8 liters per minute via face mask,
3. *discontinue* the oxytocic drug if it is being given,
4. *increase* the intravenous flow rate (if the patient has an IV) to increase circulatory volume,
5. *elevate* the patient's legs to increase blood volume in the central circulation,
6. *notify* the physician, and
7. DO NOT LEAVE THE PATIENT ALONE.

Occasionally a patient may exhibit signs of an allergic reaction to local anesthetic agents used in obstetrics. Although this is rare, it is important for the nurse to be aware of the following signs and symptoms in order to notify the physician immediately:

Mild reaction: palpitations, vertigo, tinnitus (ringing in ears), apprehension, confusion, headache, and a metallic taste in the mouth.

Moderate reaction: all of the above are intensified, with the addition of nausea and vomiting, hypotension, and muscle twitching (leading to convulsions and loss of consciousness).

Severe reaction: sudden loss of consciousness, coma, severe hypotension, bradycardia, respiratory depression, and cardiac arrest.[17]

Review Question

Following the administration of an anesthetic agent, you note that the fetal heart rate baseline has dropped to 90 to 100 beats per minute, and the patient's blood pressure has decreased significantly. List at least five emergency measures you should carry out:

a. _____

b. _____

c. _____

d. _____

e. _____

Answers

The following emergency nursing measures should be initiated: a. turn the mother on her left side, b. give oxygen at 5 to 8 liters per minute, c. discontinue oxytocic, d. increase the intravenous flow rate, e. elevate the patient's legs, f. notify the physician, and g. DO NOT LEAVE THE PATIENT ALONE.

Types of Anesthesia Used During Labor and Delivery

The chart on page 198 shows when anesthetic agents are most commonly administered during labor and delivery. The arrows denote the desired duration of action of anesthesia. Refer to this chart periodically as you read the remainder of this chapter.

The *paracervical block* is a regional anesthetic procedure that blocks nerve pathways from the uterus during labor (Figs. 7-3 and 7-4). The anesthetic agent (5 to 10 ml) is injected bilaterally into the paracervical nerve endings through the vaginal canal or transperitoneally with the patient in a lithotomy position. Novocain and Pontocaine are recommended for a paracervical block, because they are better metabolized by the placenta with less transfer to the fetus.

A paracervical block is administered during the first stage of labor (multigravida: 4 to 5 cm dilated; primigravida: 5 to 6 cm dilated) and gives complete relief of pain 80 percent of the time. The anesthetic effect is dramatic, achieved in 3 to 5 minutes and lasts 45 to 60 minutes, depending on the type and amount of agent used. The procedure may be repeated every 60 to 90 minutes as necessary. It is important to use a fetal monitor in conjunction with paracervical blocks. *Transient fetal bradycardia* may develop within 2 to 10 minutes of paracervical block administration and last 3 to 30 minutes. It is thought to be caused by

STAGE I	STAGE II	STAGE III
Paracervical Block→ (multigravida: 4–5 cm primigravida: 5–6 cm		
	Spinal Block (just prior to delivery)	——————→
	Caudal Block (just prior to delivery)	——————→
Continuous Caudal Block (6 cm)	———————————	——————→
	Lumbar Epidural Block (just prior to delivery)	——————→
Continuous Lumbar Epidural Block (6 cm)	———————————	——————→
	Pudendal Block (just prior to delivery)	——————→
	Local Perineal Block (just prior to delivery)	——————→
	Inhalation Anesthesia (immediately prior to delivery)	——————→
	Intravenous Anesthesia (immediately prior to delivery)	——————→

STAGE I—From the beginning of labor to complete dilatation of the cervix.
STAGE II—From complete dilatation through delivery of the baby.
STAGE III—From delivery of the baby through delivery of the placenta.

rapid fetal absorption of the anesthetic agent or uterine artery constriction. The previously stated interventions for fetal heart rate bradycardia are not warranted in this case.[18] However, if bradycardia persists, it is no longer considered transient and may indicate fetal distress. Although transient fetal bradycardia is considered a common side effect of paracervical blocks, this side effect could add insult to a fetus experiencing undetected distress from other causes. The paracervical block should be used *only* with normal labor and an uncompromised fetus.

The length of the needle may be frightening to the patient. The nurse should explain that the length is necessary in order to reach the cervical area. Transvaginally, the needle is inserted through a guide with

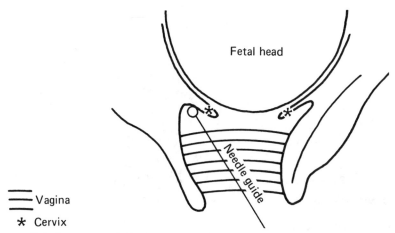

Figure 7-3. Paracervical block injection site.

only 6 to 12 mm inserted into the mucosa. The disadvantages of a paracervical block are:

1. a 2 to 70 percent incidence of fetal bradycardia,[19]
2. a decrease in labor contractions may occur for 15 minutes,
3. when the anesthetic wears off, the return of sensation is abrupt and may be interpreted as quite painful,
4. the procedure, owing to its short duration, may need to be repeated several times during labor,
5. it can only be used during the first stage of labor when the cervix is still palpable; therefore, it is not effective for delivery, and
6. if accidentally injected into the fetus it may cause apnea, bradycardia, convulsions, and central nervous system damage to the fetus.

Review Questions

1. The paracervical block is a regional anesthetic procedure used during labor to relieve pain by:

   _____

   _____

2. What nursing action should be taken immediately following administration of a paracervical block?

   _____

   _____

3. List at least three advantages of a paracervical block.

   a._____

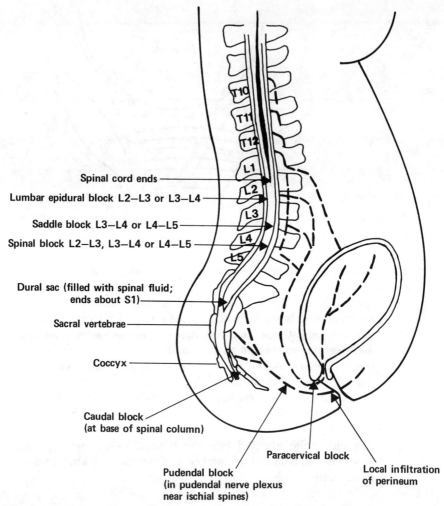

Spinal cord ends

Lumbar epidural block L2—L3 or L3—L4

Saddle block L3—L4 or L4—L5

Spinal block L2—L3, L3—L4 or L4—L5

Dural sac (filled with spinal fluid; ends about S1)

Sacral vertebrae

Coccyx

Caudal block (at base of spinal column)

Pudendal block (in pudendal nerve plexus near ischial spines)

Paracervical block

Local infiltration of perineum

Figure 7-4. Schematic drawing of the sites of anesthetic infiltration.

b. _____

c. _____

4. List at least four disadvantages of a paracervical block.

a. _____

b. _____

c. _____

d. _____

Answers

1. Paracervical blocks are used during labor to relieve pain by blocking nerve pathways from the uterus.
2. Immediately following the administration of a paracervical block the nurse should closely monitor the FHR for at least 30 minutes.
3. Advantages of a paracervical block are (a) it may be given during the first stage of labor; (b) it gives complete pain relief 80 percent of the time; (c) anesthesia is achieved in 3 to 5 minutes; and (d) it can be repeated when it wears off.
4. Disadvantages of the paracervical block are (a) transient fetal bradycardia; (b) decrease in labor contractions for 15 minutes; (c) abrupt return of pain; (d) short duration of anesthesia; (e) it is not effective for delivery; and (f) apnea, bradycardia, convulsions, and central nervous system damage to the fetus may occur if accidentally injected.

Spinal anesthesia is a broad classification of regional anesthesia brought about by injecting the anesthetic agent into the spinal canal, causing a loss of sensation below the site of injection. Spinal anesthesia includes spinal block, saddle block, and caudal and epidural blocks. The following advantages, disadvantages, and nursing care apply to *all* methods of spinal anesthesia.

Advantages of spinal anesthesia:

1. It provides anesthesia from the end of Stage I (epidurals and caudals may be given earlier) through the repair of the episiotomy.
2. It tends to prevent precipitous delivery because the urge to push is blocked, although the ability to push is present in varying degrees.
3. The mother remains awake and is able to participate in the birth experience.
4. There are no direct side effects on the fetus or newborn, unless the fetus is accidentally injected with the anesthetic agent.

Disadvantages of spinal anesthesia:

1. The most common side effect is maternal hypotension, causing decreased oxygenation to the fetus. Any decrease in maternal blood pressure is probably associated with an equal decrease in placental blood flow.[20] Prevention of maternal hypotension may be achieved by (1) IV fluid hydration of the mother prior to administration of the anesthetic agent;[21] and (2) positioning the mother on her side during labor or using the left lateral tilt

position during delivery. This helps avoid supine hypotension syndrome.[22] (See Chapter 1.)

2. The mother's decreased urge to push usually decreases pushing effectiveness, necessitating the use of forceps to facilitate the delivery. (There is an increased incidence of persistent occiput posterior and occiput transverse positions[23] with the use of spinal anesthesia.)

3. Owing to increased pressure in the epidural and subarachnoid spaces during labor contractions, injection of anesthetic agents must be done between contractions to prevent excessively high anesthesia levels.[24]

4. Some patients may develop a postspinal headache due to a loss of spinal fluid through a puncture of the dura (spinal block and saddle block). The incidence of postspinal headache is only 2 percent when a small (25 to 26-gauge) needle is used for the procedure.[25] Bed rest after a dural puncture does not reduce the incidence of spinal headache;[26] however, many physicians still order that the patient be kept flat 4 to 12 hours after delivery.

5. It may cause uterine contractions to decrease in frequency and intensity. If labor fails to progress, oxytocin augmentation may be necessary.

6. It causes decreased sensitivity to the filling urinary bladder (beyond the normal decreased sensitivity) so that some patients need to be catheterized after delivery to prevent bladder distention which may cause postpartum hemorrhage.

General nursing care of the patient receiving spinal anesthesia includes:

1. helping the patient maintain the desired position during administration of the anesthetic (positions for each procedure will be discussed later);

2. providing emotional support;

3. continually monitoring contraction patterns, blood pressure, pulse, and fetal heart rate;

4. evaluating bladder status: a full bladder may impede the labor and delivery process and cause trauma to the bladder;

5. instructing and coaching for effective pushing during Stage II;

6. and during the postpartum period, checking for bladder distention, fundal consistency and placement, and return of sensation to the lower extremities.

Review Questions

1. Is spinal anesthesia classified as regional or local? _____

2. List at least three advantages of spinal anesthesia.
   a. _____
   b. _____
   c. _____

3. List at least three disadvantages of spinal anesthesia.
   a. _____
   b. _____
   c. _____

4. List at least three nursing responsibilities related to the administration of spinal anesthesia.
   a. _____
   b. _____
   c. _____

Answers

1. Spinal anesthesia is classified as *regional*.
2. Advantages of spinal anesthesia are: (a) it provides anesthesia during Stages I, II, and III; (b) it tends to prevent precipitous delivery; (c) the mother is able to participate in the birth experience; and (d) there are no direct side effects on the fetus or newborn.
3. Disadvantages of spinal anesthesia are (a) maternal hypotension, causing decreased oxygenation of the fetus; (b) the mother's decreased urge to push causes increased use of forceps for delivery; (c) anesthetic injection into the epidural and subarachnoid spaces must be done between contractions; (d) loss of spinal fluid may cause postspinal headache; (e) it may interrupt labor progression necessitating oxytocin augmentation; and (f) after delivery, bladder catheterization may be necessary to prevent postpartum hemorrhage.
4. Nursing responsibilities related to the administration of spinal anesthesia include (a) helping the patient maintain the desired position during administration of the anesthetic; (b) providing emotional support; (c) continually monitoring contractions, blood pressure, pulse, and fetal heart rate; (d) evaluating bladder status; (e) instructing and coaching effective pushing; and (f) during the immediate postpartum period, checking for bladder distention, fundal consistency and placement, and return of sensation to the lower extremities.

The *spinal block*[27] or subarachnoid block (Fig. 7-4) is a regional anesthetic used just prior to delivery. A hyperbaric (heavier than spinal fluid) anesthetic solution is injected into the subarachnoid space between the dura and the spinal canal. This cavity is filled with cerebrospinal fluid.

The site of injection is the space between L-2 and L-3, L-3 and L-4, or L-4 and L-5. The patient may be in a sitting or side-lying position (Sims).

Spinal block for cesarean delivery requires blockage of impulses to the level of T-6. This provides anesthesia from the nipple line to the toes. (Anesthesia levels above T-4 will stop respiratory function.) In order to achieve a high level of anesthesia, dosage of the agent and patient position are important. The patient is placed in a supine position immediately after administration of the block.

A low spinal block (to the level of T-10) provides complete relief of pain for a vaginal delivery with loss of sensation from the umbilicus to the toes. A smaller amount of anesthetic is used and the patient remains sitting for 30 seconds to 1 minute before being placed in a supine position. A low spinal block is sometimes inappropriately called a saddle block.

The true *saddle block*[28] (Fig. 7-4) is a specific type of spinal block, not a different type of block. Those parts of the saddle (perineum, lower pelvis, and upper thighs) are anesthetized by blocking nerves from S-1 to S-4. The anesthetic agent is injected into the subarachnoid space. The site of injection is the space between L-3 and L-4 or L-4 and L-5. Following injection, the patient remains sitting for 3 to 5 minutes to insure a low level of anesthesia. Pain relief for delivery is not complete, because only the sacral nerves are blocked; however, the patient is able to push more effectively with a saddle block than with a low spinal block.

The *caudal block* (Fig. 7-4) is a regional spinal anesthetic affecting the entire pelvic area. Therefore, the patient does not feel uterine contractions or perineal stretching during the delivery. The amount of anesthetic agent injected will determine the level of anesthesia achieved. For a vaginal delivery, blockage of T-10 to L-1 will provide anesthesia from the umbilicus to midthigh. The anesthetic agent is injected into the caudal space of the sacral canal which is level with the last sacral vertebra. This is a potential space surrounding the dura and does not contain cerebrospinal fluid. The caudal block is administered during the second stage of labor just prior to delivery, with the patient in a Sims or knee-chest position. A disadvantage of caudal anesthesia is that accidental injection of the fetus may cause apnea, bradycardia, convulsions, and central nervous system damage.

The *continuous caudal block* is the same as the caudal block except that it provides anesthesia during Stages I through III. By inserting a polyethylene tubing into the caudal space when approximately 6 cm dilatation is reached, the effect of anesthesia may be maintained through repeated injections of the anesthetic agent into the tubing as necessary (every 45 to 90 minutes).

The *lumbar epidural block*[27] (Fig. 7-4) is a regional anesthesia affecting the entire pelvis by blocking nerve impulses at the level of T-12 through S-5. Blockage of T-10 through L-1 provides anesthesia from the umbilicus to midthigh, rendering complete relief of pain for vaginal delivery. With the patient in a Sims or sitting position, the anesthetic agent is injected into the epidural space (the space surrounding the dura) which lies between the dura mater and the ligamentum flavum. The site of entry is the space between L-2 and L-3 or L-3 and L-4.

Cesarean delivery may be accomplished with an epidural block; however, anesthesia must block nerves from T-7 to L-5. This level provides anesthesia from the nipple line to the toes. Movement and pressure may be felt but no pain. The patient may need reassurance, since she may feel that her ability to breathe adequately is decreased.

The major complication of epidural anesthesia is dural puncture (the needle is inserted beyond the dura mater into the spinal canal) which causes spinal block anesthesia. Depending on the site of insertion and the amount of anesthetic agent, this accidental puncture of the dura with injection of anesthetic agents into the subarachnoid space may cause severe hypotension, coma, and respiratory arrest.

Lumbar epidural block using Marcaine as the anesthetic agent has been reported to produce undesirable side effects in the newborn which include muscular hypotonia, diminished Moro reflex, occasional behavioral alterations, and decreased motor activity.[27]

The *continuous lumbar epidural block* is the same as the lumbar epidural block except that it provides continuous anesthesia during Stages I through III. It may be introduced at 6 cm dilatation and maintained through a polyethylene tubing as in the continuous caudal block. It is commonly believed that labor progression will be decreased if the epidural block is administered prior to 5 cm dilatation. There is little evidence to support this belief.[29,30]

Spinal anesthesia is used primarily to achieve anesthesia of the pelvic area. However, varying degrees of temporary loss of sensation to the lower extremities may also occur. The duration of anesthesia to the lower extremities varies according to the drug used, the dosage, and the route of administration. It is important to be aware of these factors while positioning the patient on the delivery table and removing her legs from the stirrups to prevent damage. Ambulation should not be attempted until full sensation has returned.

Review Question

The following are regional block anesthetics. Prior to a vaginal delivery identify for each type the location of injection, spinal nerves blocked, area of anesthesia desired, position of the patient, stage in labor when used, and the most common side effects.

Name	Location	Spinal nerves affected	Area of anesthesia	Position	Stage	Most common side effects
Spinal block						
Saddle block						
Caudal block						
Lumbar epidural block						

Answer

Prior to a vaginal delivery for each type of regional anesthetic, the location of injection, spinal nerves blocked, area of anesthesia, position of the patient, stage in labor used and the most common side effects are:

Name	Location	Spinal nerves affected	Area of anesthesia	Position	Stage	Most common side effects
Spinal block	Subarachnoid space L2-L3; L3-L4, or L4-L5	T10-L5	Umbilicus to toes	Sims or sitting	II	Headache; maternal hypotension
Saddle block	Subarachnoid space L3-L4 or L4-L5	S1-S4	Perineum, lower pelvis, and upper thighs	Sims or sitting	II	Headache; maternal hypotension
Caudal block	Caudal space of the sacral canal	T10-L1	Umbilicus to midthigh	Sims or knee-chest	I, II	Maternal hypotension
Lumbar epidural block	Epidural space surrounding the dura L2-L3 or L3-L4	T10-L1	Umbilicus to midthigh	Sims or sitting	I, II	Maternal hypotension

The *pudendal block* (Fig. 7-4) is a form of local anesthesia that provides anesthesia to the perineal area, vulva, and vagina. The block interferes with impulses from S-2 to S-4 by injection of the anesthetic agent into the pudendal nerve endings at the ischial spine level (bilaterally). The block is administered just prior to delivery through the vaginal wall with the patient in a lithotomy position. The onset of action is immediate, with a duration of 30 minutes. Anesthesia should allow delivery and episiotomy repair without pain. The pudendal block may be the anesthesia of choice for a delivery following the use of paracervical blocks during the first stage of labor. Complications are not common but may include sciatic nerve damage, broad ligament hematoma, and perforation of the rectum.

Advantages of the pudendal block:
1. It produces marked relaxation of perineal muscles, facilitating an easier delivery with decreased possibility of perineal tears.
2. The mother is still able to push effectively, although the urge to push is slightly diminished.
3. There are seldom side effects in the fetus or newborn, unless it is accidentally injected with the anesthetic agent.

Disadvantages of the pudendal block:
1. The mother may still experience pain with contractions and stretching of the vaginal wall during delivery and placental expulsion.

The *local perineal infiltration* (Fig. 7-4) is a local anesthesia sometimes used in conjunction with other regional anesthetics if necessary. Just prior to delivery, medication is injected locally into the perineal body to desensitize the episiotomy site. Nesacaine, Xylocaine, and Carbocaine are most commonly used because of their rapid tissue diffusion.

Advantages of local perineal infiltration:
1. The mother is able to push effectively and cooperate in the delivery of the baby.
2. There are no side effects on the fetus or newborn.
3. It provides effective anesthesia for cutting and repair of the episiotomy.

Disadvantages of local perineal infiltration:
1. It does not eliminate pain or discomfort from perineal distention, contractions, or placental expulsion.
2. Used alone, it is usually only effective for the episiotomy repair.

Review Questions

1. The pudendal block is used to block nerve endings at the _____ _____ to provide relaxation of _____ and anesthesia of the _____ .

2. List at least two advantages of the pudendal block.

    a. _____

    b. _____

3. Give one disadvantage of the pudendal block.

    _____

    _____

4. Local perineal infiltration is used just prior to delivery to desensitize
    the _____ .

5. List at least two advantages of local perineal infiltration.

    a. _____

    b. _____

Answers

1. The pudendal block is used to block nerve endings at the *ischial
    spine level* to provide relaxation of *perineal muscles* and anesthesia
    of the *perineum*.

2. Advantages of the pudendal block are (a) it produces marked relax-
    ation of the perineum facilitating an easier delivery with decreased
    possibility of perineal tears; (b) the mother is still able to push
    effectively, although the urge is slightly diminished; (c) there are
    seldom side effects on the fetus or newborn unless it is accidentally
    injected with the anesthetic agent.

3. A disadvantage of the pudendal block is that the mother may still
    experience pain with contractions and stretching of the vaginal wall
    during delivery and placental expulsion.

4. Local perineal infiltration is used just prior to delivery to desensitize
    the *episiotomy site*.

5. Advantages of local perineal infiltration are (a) the mother is able
    to push effectively and cooperate in the delivery of the baby; (b)
    there are no side effects on the fetus or newborn; and (c) it provides
    effective anesthesia for cutting and repair of the episiotomy.

Inhalation anesthesia is not prevalent today for normal deliveries. It
is sometimes used for cesarean births, although spinal or lumbar epidural
anesthesia is frequently used. The agent of choice (nitrous oxide) is
combined with oxygen and inhaled through a mask in gaseous form to
provide anesthesia of the entire body and loss of consciousness. It is
important to deliver the baby within 5 to 7 minutes after administration
of the gas, because inhalation anesthesia rapidly crosses the placenta to

the fetus resulting in anoxia and respiratory depression of the fetus or newborn. Inhalation anesthesia produces depression of the central nervous system; therefore, it is important to continually monitor maternal vital signs before, during, and after administration of the anesthetic. Continual fetal heart rate monitoring is essential prior to delivery followed by Apgar scoring and assessment of the newborn immediately after delivery. Advantages of inhalation anesthesia:

1. It produces greater overall body muscle relaxation (it especially facilitates cesarean births).
2. It causes a decreased possibility of toxemic convulsions, because it depresses the central nervous system. This may be the anesthetic of choice for the mother with severe toxemia of pregnancy.

Disadvantages of inhalation anesthesia:

1. Rapid placental diffusion of anesthesia causes fetal anesthesia with respiratory depression and anoxia of the newborn.
2. Increased possibility of maternal aspiration of gastric contents may cause pneumonia or even death.
3. The mother is unable to participate in the delivery.
4. The father's presence at the delivery is usually undesirable.
5. A trained anesthetist or anesthesiologist must be present to administer the agent.
6. Recovery period for the mother is longer, with postpartum nausea and vomiting often present.
7. The mother must be assessed carefully for postpartum hemorrhage due to the uterine relaxant effect of nitrous oxide.

Intravenous anesthesia is rarely seen in modern obstetrics. Sodium pentothal (a short-acting barbiturate) is injected into the blood stream, causing a loss of sensation to the entire body and a loss of consciousness. It causes rapid induction of anesthesia and prompt recovery. Constant monitoring of vital signs is imperative.

Major disadvantages of intravenous anesthesia:

1. Maternal bronchospasms and laryngospasms may lead to respiratory arrest.
2. Indirect fetal hypoxia may result from maternal hypotension.

Review Questions

1. When administering inhalation anesthesia for a delivery, the most important consideration is _____
   _____
   _____

2. List two advantages of inhalation anesthesia.
   a. _____
   b. _____

210

3. List at least five disadvantages of inhalation anesthesia.
   a. _____
   b. _____
   c. _____
   d. _____
   e. _____

4. The drug most commonly used for intravenous anesthesia is
   _____

5. List two complications of intravenous anesthesia.
   a. _____
   b. _____

Answers

1. When administering inhalation anesthesia for delivery, the most important consideration is *the amount of time between the onset of administration and the birth of the baby.*

2. Advantages of inhalation anesthesia are (a) greater overall body muscle relaxation; (b) decreased possibility of toxemic convulsions due to central nervous system depression.

3. Disadvantages of inhalation anesthesia are (a) rapid placental diffusion of anesthesia, causing fetal anesthesia with respiratory depression and anoxia of the newborn; (b) increased possibility of maternal aspiration of gastric contents, causing pneumonia or even death; (c) no participation in the delivery by the mother; (d) makes father's presence at the delivery undesirable; (e) a trained anesthetist must be present to administer the agent; (f) recovery period for the mother is longer, with postpartum nausea and vomiting often present; and (g) uterine relaxation causing postpartum hemorrhage may occur.

4. *Sodium pentothal* is most commonly used for intravenous anesthesia.

5. Complications of intravenous anesthesia are (a) maternal bronchospasms and laryngospasms that may lead to respiratory arrest; and (b) indirect fetal hypoxia due to maternal hypotension.

In conclusion, the process of labor and delivery is considered a maturational crisis to which patients respond in a variety of ways. If the patient is unprepared for the experience, she may interpret the contractions of labor as being excessively painful. Excessive pain can be detrimental; therefore, the cycle must be interrupted through the careful and proper use of analgesics, anesthetics, and supportive nursing interventions. Drugs given to a woman in labor affect not only her but may also have undesirable indirect effects upon the fetus or newborn. What to give and when to give it can sometimes be a very difficult decision to make. Ideally, the woman who is able to progress normally through the process of labor and delivery should be given as little medication as possible. *Perhaps, none at all may be best.*

REFERENCES

1.. AKAMATSU, TJ AND BONICA, JJ: *Pain pathway during labor.* IN CLARK, AL AND AFFONSO, DD: *Childbearing: A Nursing Perspective,* ed 2. FA Davis, Philadelphia, 1979, p 421.

2. MCCAFFERY, M: *Nursing Management of the Patient With Pain,* ed 2, JB Lippincott, Philadelphia, 1979, p 63.

3. SHNIDER, SM AND MOYA, F: *Effects of meperidine on the newborn infant.* Am J Obstet Gynecol 89:1009, 1964.

4. BRACKBILL, Y, ET AL: *Obstetric premedication and infant outcome.* Am J Obstet Gynecol 118:377, 1974.

5. STECHLER, G: *Newborn attention as affected by medication during labor.* Science 144:315, 1964.

6. HODGKINSON, R ET AL: *Neonatal neurobehavior in the first 48 hours of life: Effect of the administration of meperidine with and without Naloxone in the mother.* Pediatrics 62(3):297, 1978.

7. KRON, RE, STEIN, M, AND GODDARD, DE: *Newborn sucking behavior affected by obstetric sedation.* Pediatrics 37:1012, 1966.

8. BORGSTEDT, AD, AND ROSEN, MG: *Medication during labor correlated with behavior and EEG of the newborn.* Am J Dis Child 115:21, 1968.

9. FLOWERS, CE AND RUDOLPH AJ: *Diazepam (Valium) as an adjunct in obstetric analgesia.* Obstet Gynecol 34:68, 1969.

10. SCOTT, DB: *Analgesia in labor.* Br J Anaesth 69:11, 1977.

11. FINSTER, M, ET AL: *Reassessment of the metabolism of 2-Chloroprocaine HC1 (Nesacaine).* ASA Abstracts pp 29–30, 1973.

12. SCANLON, NJ, ET AL: *Neurobehavioral responses and drug concentrations in newborns after maternal epidural anesthesia with bupivacaine.* Anesthesiology 45:400, 1976.

13. TUCKER, GT, ET AL: *Binding amilide-type local anesthetics in human plasma II.* Anesthesiology 33:304, 1970.

14. BROWN, WU, JR, ET AL: *Newborn levels of lidocaine and mepivacaine in the first post natal day following maternal epidural anesthesia.* Anesthesiology 42:698, 1975.

15. SCANLON, JW, ET AL: *Neurobehavioral responses of newborn infants after maternal epidural anesthesia.* Anesthesiology 40:121, 1974.

16. MOORE, DC, ET AL: *Accumulation of mepivicaine HC1 during caudal block.* Anesthesiology 29:585, 1968.

17. OLDS, SB, ET AL: *Obstetric Nursing.* Addison-Wesley, Menlo Park California, 1980, p 533.

18. RALSTON, DH AND SHNIDER, SM: *The fetal and neonatal effects of regional anesthesia in obstetrics.* Anesthesiology 48(1):34, 1978.

19. KING, JC AND SHERLINE, DM: *Paracervical and pudendal block.* Clin Obstet Gynecol 24(2):590, 1981.

20. GREISS, FC: *A clinical concept of uterine blood flow during pregnancy.* Obstet Gynecol 30:595, 1967.

21. WOLLMAN, SB AND MARX, GF: *Acute hydration for prevention of hypotension and spinal anesthesia in parturients.* Anesthesiology 29:374, 1968.

22. Clark, RB: *Prevention and treatment of aortocaval compression in the pregnant patient.* Anesth Rev 7:13, 1980.

23. HOULT, IJ, MACLENNAN, AH, AND CARRIE, LES: *Lumbar epidural analgesia in labour. Relation to foetal malposition and instrumental delivery.* Br Med J 3:114, 1977.

24. FULBERT, MN AND MARX, GF: *Extradural pressures in the parturient patient.* Anesthesiology 40:499, 1974.

25. GREENE, BA: *A 26-gauge lumbar puncture needle: Its value in the prophylaxis of headache following spinal analgesia for vaginal delivery.* Anesthesiology 11:464, 1950.

26. JONES, RJ: *The role of recumbency in the prevention and treatment of postspinal headache.* Anesth Analg 53:788, 1974.

27. ROSENBLATT, DB, ET AL: *The influence of maternal analgesia on neonatal behavior: II. Epidural bupivacaine.* Br J Obstet Gynaecol 88:407, 1981.

28. CLARK, RB: *Conduction anesthesia.* Clin Obstet Gynecol 24(2):603, 1981.

29. PHILLIPS, JC, ET AL: *Epidural analgesia and its effects on the "normal" progress of labor.* Am J Obstet Gynecol 129:316, 1977.

30. CRAWFORD, JS: *The second thousand epidural blocks in an obstetric hospital practice.* Br J Anaesth 46:1277, 1972.

BIBLIOGRAPHY

BARAKA, A, NOUEIHIB, R, AND HAJJ, S: *Intrathecal injection of morphine for obstetric analgesia.* Anesthesiology 54(2):136, 1981.

BELSEY, EM, ET AL: *The influence of maternal analgesia on neonatal behavior: I. Pethidine.* Br J Obstet Gynaecol 88:398, 1981.

BONICA, J: *Principles and Practice of Obstetric Analgesia and Anesthesia.* FA Davis, Philadelphia, 1972.

CLARK, AL AND AFFONSO, DD: *Childbearing: A Nursing Perspective,* ed 2. FA Davis, Philadelphia, 1979.

CLARK, RB: *Conduction anesthesia.* Clin Obstet Gynecol 24(2):601, 1981.

CRAWFORD, JS: *Continuous lumbar epidural analgesia for labour and delivery.* Br Med J 1(6156):72, 1979.

DILTS, PV: *Narcotic analgesia.* Clin Obstet Gynecol 24(2):597, 1981.

ENDLER, JC: *Conduction anesthesia in obstetrics and its effects upon fetus and newborn.* J Reprod Med 24:83, 1980.

FLOYD, CC: *Drugs for childbirth: Your guide to their risks and benefits.* R.N. 5:41, 1977.

FOX, HS: *The effects of catecholamines and drug treatment on the fetus and newborn.* Birth and the Family Journal 6(3):157, 1979.

GRAD, RK AND WOODSIDE, J: *Obstetrical analgesics and anesthesia: Methods of relief for the patient in labor.* Am J Nurs 77(2)242, 1977.

HILL, RM AND BARTON, MD: *Maternal drugs in the prenatal and intrapartal period and their effect on the neonate. Perinatal Pharmacology.* Mead Johnson Symposium on Perinatal and Developmental Medicine 5:39, 1974.

HODGKINSON, R, ET AL: *Neonatal neurobehavior in the first 48 hours of life: Effect of the administration of meperidine with and without naloxone in the mother.* Pediatrics 62(3):294, 1978.

JENSON, MD, BENSON, RC, AND BOBAK, IM: *Maternity Care: The Nurse and the Family,* ed 2. CV Mosby, St. Louis, 1981.

KING, JC AND SHERLINE, DM: *Paracervical and pudendal block.* Clin Obstet Gynecol 24(2):587, 1981.

KRON, RE, ET AL: *Newborn sucking behavior affected by obstetric sedation.* Pediatrics 37(6):1012, 1966.

KUHNERT, BR, ET AL: *Meperidine and normeperidine levels following meperidine administration during labor: I. Mother.* Am J Obstet Gynecol 133(8):904, 1979.

KUHNERT, BR, ET AL: *Meperidine and normeperidine levels following meperidine administration during labor: II. Fetus and Neonate.* Am J Obstet Gynecol 133(8):909, 1979.

LEVINSON, G AND SHNIDER, SM: *Catecholamines: The effects of maternal fear and its treatment on uterine function and circulation.* Birth and the Family Journal 6(3):167, 1979.

LIEBERMAN, BA, ET AL: *The effects of maternally administered pethidine or epidural bupivacaine on the fetus and newborn.* Br J Obstet Gynaecol 86:598, 1979.

McCAFFERY, J: *Nursing Management of the Patient With Pain,* ed 2. JB Lippincott, Philadelphia, 1979.

McDONALD, JS: *Obstetric Anesthesia.* Clin Obstet Gynecol 21:489, 1978.

McLAUGHLIN, SM AND TAUBENHEIM, AM: *Epidural anesthesia for obstetric patients.* J Obstet Gynecol Neonatal Nurs 10(1):9, 1981.

MERKOW, AJ, ET AL: *The neonatal neurobehavioral effects of bupivacaine, mepivacaine and 2-chloroprocaine used for pudendal block.* Anesthesiology 52(4):309, 1980.

MORGAN, BM, REHOR, S, AND LEWIS, PJ: *Epidural analgesia for uneventful labour.* Anesthesia 35(1):57, 1980.

MOZINGO, JN: *Pain in labor: A conceptual model for intervention.* J Obstet Gynecol Neonatal Nurs 7:47, 1978.

Obstetrical Analgesia and Anesthesia. PITKIN, R AND ZLATNIK, F (EDS): *The Year Book of OB GYN 1980.* Year Book Medical Publishers, Chicago, 1980.

OLDS, SB, ET AL: *Obstetric Nursing.* Addison-Wesley, Menlo Park California, 1981.

PILLITTERI, A: *Maternal-Newborn Nursing: Care of the Growing Family,* ed 2. Little, Brown & Co, Boston, 1981.

PRITCHARD, JA AND MCDONALD, PC: *William's Obstetrics,* ed 15. Appleton-Century-Crofts, New York, 1976.

REISNER, LS: *Anesthesia for cesarean section.* Clin Obstet Gynecol 23(2)517, 1980.

ROSENBLATT, DB ET AL: *The influence of maternal analgesia on neonatal behaviour: II. Epidural bupivacaine.* Br J Obstet Gynaecol 88:407, 1981.

SCANLON, JW: *Obstetric anesthesia as a neonatal risk factor in normal labor and delivery.* Clin Perinatol 1(2):465, 1974.

SCANLON, NJ, ET AL: *Neurobehavioral responses and drug concentrations in newborn after maternal epidural anesthesia with bupivacaine.* Anesthesiology 45:400, 1976.

SCANLON, JW: *Effects of obstetric anesthesia and analgesia on the newborn: A select, annotated bibliography for the clinician.* Clin Obstet Gynecol 24(2):649, 1981.

SHNIDER, SM AND MOYA, F: *Effects of meperidine on the newborn infant.* Am J Obstet Gynecol 89:1009, 1961.

The Risks of Paracervical Anesthesia Intoxication and Neurological Injury of the Newborn. Pediatrics 55(4):533, 1975.

TRONICK, F, ET AL: *Regional obstetric anesthesia and newborn behavior: Effect over the first ten days of life.* Pediatrics 58:94, 1976.

WIENER, PC, HOGG, MI AND ROSEN, M: *Neonatal respiration, feeding and neurobehavioural state: Effects of intrapartum bupivacaine, pethidine and pethidine reversed by naloxone.* Anesthesia 34:996, 1979.

POST-TEST

1. Pain is a subjective phenomenon that exists when an individual:
   a. _____
   b. _____
   c. _____
2. Differentiate among the following factors that may accompany an individual's reaction to pain as: (a) physiologic, (b) verbal, or (c) nonverbal. Place the appropriate letter (a, b, or c) in front of each descriptive term.
   _____ (1) depression   _____ (9) increased muscle
   _____ (2) increased BP   tension
   _____ (3) moaning   _____ (10) hostility
   _____ (4) rigidity   _____ (11) groaning

_____ (5) grimacing   _____ (12) increased respirations

_____ (6) fear   _____ (13) pacing

_____ (7) dilated pupils   _____ (14) withdrawal

_____ (8) cries for help

3. List at least four reasons why pain may occur during labor.

a._____

b. _____

c. _____

d. _____

4. What is analgesia? What is the most common analgesic drug used in labor?_____

_____

_____

5. What desirable effects should analgesia have on the mother? What is the major undesirable effect?_____

_____

_____

6. How might analgesia administered to the mother indirectly affect the fetus? What nursing interventions are appropriate? How might it affect the newborn?_____

_____

_____

_____

7. What subtle behavioral changes have been observed in the newborn during the first 24 hours of life following the use of Demerol for the mother during labor?_____

_____

_____

How might the new mother feel about these behavioral changes in the newborn?_____

_____

_____

What are the appropriate nursing interventions?_____

_____

_____

8. What three factors must be carefully considered when deciding on a program of drug intervention for the woman in labor?

a. _____

b. _____

c. _____

9. Name the direct maternal effects of drug intervention that can indirectly affect the fetus or newborn.
   a. _____
   b. _____
   c. _____
10. What can the nurse do, in addition to providing medication, to decrease a patient's perception of pain?
    a. _____
    b. _____
    c. _____
    d. _____
    e. _____
11. Key: A. Demerol
          B. Barbiturates
          C. Scopolamine
          D. Tranquilizers
          E. Narcotic antagonists

The following statements need to be completed. Insert the appropriate letter (using the above key) to make the statements correct.

(a) _____ may be given alone in early labor to decrease apprehension and anxiety, promote sedation, and relieve nausea.

(b) _____ Respiratory depression is the *major* side effect of ____ _____ .

(c) _____ Although sedation is the desired effect, _____ _____ may cause disorientation with marked excitement and delirium.

(d) _____ When _____ is administered to the mother during labor, subtle behavioral changes may be observed in the newborn during the first 24 hours of life.

(e) _____ During the first 4 days of life, the newborn may exhibit poor sucking reflex, fewer sucks per minute, lower sucking pressure and decreased formula intake when _____have been administered to the mother during labor.

(f) _____ Respiratory depression of the newborn caused by barbiturates, tranquilizers, and sedatives may be increased when _____ _____ are administered.

(g) _____ The attention span of the newborn after birth is thought to be affected by maternal administration of _____ _____ during labor.

(h) _____ Newborn hypothermia and hypotonia are thought to be caused by intrapartal administration of _____ .

(j) _____ Maternal hypotension is the major side effect of _____
_____ drugs.

(j) _____ _____ administered at the appropriate time in labor may promote cervical relaxation,
thereby enhancing labor progression.

12. Since anesthetic agents might cause maternal hypotension or fetal
bradycardia, what five nursing actions would be appropriate if one
or both did occur?
a. _____
b. _____
c. _____
d. _____
e. _____

13. Key: A. Paracervical
         B. Spinal
         C. Saddle
         D. Epidural
         E. Pudendal
         F. Local

The following statements need to be completed. Insert the appropriate
letter (using the above key) to make the statements correct.

(a) _____ The episiotomy site is desensitized just prior to delivery with _____ .

(b) _____ A puncture through the dura into the subarachnoid
space is necessary for administration of _____
_____ and _____ .

(c) _____ Dural puncture is the major complication of _____
_____ .

(d) _____ Transient fetal bradycardia is the major side effect of
_____ .

(e) _____ Although the urge to push is slightly diminished, the
mother is able to push effectively following _____
_____ .

(f) _____ The space that is level with the last sacral vertebra is
the site of injection for _____ .

(g) _____ A continuous anesthetic effect during labor and delivery can be obtained with _____
and _____ .

(h) _____ _____ is used to block nerves at
the ischial spine level to provide anesthesia to the
perineal area, vulva, and vagina.

(i) _____ A headache is a side effect of _____
and _____ .

(j) _____ The major side effect of maternal hypotension is associated with _____ , _____
_____ , _____ , and
_____ anesthesia.
(k) _____ The _____ is effective only during Stage I of labor.
(l) _____ The _____ provides anesthesia to the perineum, lower pelvis, and upper thighs only.
(m) _____ _____ anesthesia is administered into the space surrounding the dura between L2-L3 or L3-L4.

ANSWERS

1. Pain is a subjective phenomenon that exists when an individual: (a) experiences a sensation; (b) interprets the sensation as painful; and (c) exhibits a psychologic and physiologic reaction to the sensation.
2. (1) c; (2) a; (3) b; (4) a; (5) a; (6) c; (7) a; (8) b; (9) a; (10) c; (11) b; (12) a; (13) a; (14) c.
    Physiologic reactions to pain include increased blood pressure, heart rate, respirations, pupil diameter, muscle tension, and muscle activity.
    Verbal reactions to pain include cries for help, moaning, and groaning.
    Nonverbal reactions to pain include depression, hostility, fear, and withdrawal.
3. The following are theories of the causes of pain in labor:
    a. Anoxia of compressed muscle cells of the uterus brought about with each contraction.
    b. Compression of the nerve ganglia in the cervix and lower uterine segments during contractions.
    c. Stretching of the cervix during dilatation and effacement.
    d. Stretching and displacing of the perineum as the fetus descends the birth canal.
    e. Pressure on the urethra, bladder, and rectum as the fetus descends.
    f. Fear resulting in tension causing pain and more fear as a spontaneous occurrence.
4. Analgesia is the absence or decreased awareness of a normal sensation of pain. The narcotic Demerol is the most common analgesic used in labor.
5. The desirable effects of analgesia upon the mother are relief of pain, antispasmodic action, decreased anxiety, euphoria, and sedation. The major undesirable effect is that it may cause respiratory depression.

6. Narcotics administered to the mother in labor may cause respiratory depression of the fetus. No specific nursing intervention is required as long as placental sufficiency is maintained for adequate oxygenation of the fetus. However, at birth, if the newborn exhibits signs of narcotic depression, resuscitative measures will be necessary.

7. Demerol administered to the mother during labor may produce subtle behavioral changes in the newborn during the first 24 hours of life. These newborns tend to be less alert and generally demonstrate sluggish behavior. They exhibit a decreased response to maternal stimuli such as startling, cuddling, and consoling. The nurse should try to help the new mother understand that the newborn will become more alert and responsive with time. She needs much assurance that the unresponsiveness of her baby is not a reflection of her mothering ability.

8. Three important considerations regarding drug intervention are:
   a. potency of the drug,
   b. side effects on the mother and fetus/newborn,
   c. stage in labor and progress made.

9. Direct maternal effects of drug intervention may cause the following indirect effects on the fetus or newborn:
   a. impaired maternal ventilation or arterial hypotension can cause decreased fetal heart rate;
   b. maternal arterial hypertension can cause abruption of the placenta with fetal anoxia and possible death;
   c. alteration in the forces of labor can cause fetal trauma due to prolonged labor.

10. In addition to providing medication, the nurse can help decrease the patient's perception of pain by:
    a. teaching or reinforcing relaxation techniques;
    b. encouraging comfortable and appropriate breathing patterns throughout labor;
    c. praising positive efforts made by the couple;
    d. promoting rest between contractions;
    e. informing the couple of effective progress throughout labor;
    f. accurately assessing reactions to pain and need for analgesia;
    g. assessing the effectiveness of analgesics when used, without losing sight of possible side effects.

11. The following statements are correct.
    (a) D; (b) A; (c) C; (d) A; (e) B; (f) E; (g) D; (h) D; (i) D; (j) A.
    (a) *Tranquilizers* may be given alone in early labor to decrease apprehension and anxiety, promote sedation, and relieve nausea.
    (b) Respiratory depression is the major side effect of *Demerol*.
    (c) Although sedation is the desired effect, *Scopolamine* may cause disorientation with marked excitement and delirium.

(d) When *Demerol* is administered to the mother during labor subtle behavioral changes may be observed in the newborn during the first 24 hours of life.

(e) During the first 4 days of life, the newborn may exhibit poor sucking reflex, fewer sucks per minute, lower sucking pressure, and decreased formula intake when *Barbiturates* have been administered to the mother during labor.

(f) Depression from barbiturates, tranquilizers, and sedatives may be increased when *Narcotic Antagonists* are administered.

(g) The attention span of the newborn after birth is thought to be affected by maternal administration of *Tranquilizers (Phenergan)* during labor.

(h) Newborn hypothermia and hypotonia are thought to be caused by the intrapartal administration of *Tranquilizers (Valium)*.

(i) Maternal hypotension is the major side effect of *Tranquilizers*.

(j) *Demerol* administered at the appropriate time in labor may promote cervical relaxation, thereby enhancing labor progression.

12. If maternal hypotension or fetal bradycardia occurs following anesthetic administration, the following nursing actions are appropriate.

a. Turn the mother on her left side to relieve uterine pressure on the iliac veins and inferior vena cava, and promote venous return, thereby increasing oxygen supply to the fetus.

b. Administer oxygen at 5 to 8 liters per minute via face mask.

c. Discontinue oxytocic drug.

d. Increase the intravenous flow rate to increase circulatory volume.

e. Elevate the patient's legs to increase blood volume in the central circulation.

f. Notify the physician.

g. DO NOT LEAVE THE PATIENT ALONE.

13. The following statements are correct.
(a) G; (b) B and C; (c) E; (d) A; (e) F; (f) D; (g) D and E; (h) F; (i) B and C; (j) B, C, D, and E; (k) A; (l) C; (m) E

(a) The episiotomy site is desensitized just prior to delivery with *Local*.

(b) A puncture through the dura into the subarachnoid space is necessary for administration of *Spinal* and *Saddle*.

(c) Dural puncture is the major complication of *Epidural*.

(d) Transient fetal bradycardia is the major side effect of *Paracervical*.

(e) Although the urge to push is slightly diminished, the mother is able to push effectively following *Pudendal*.

(f) The space that is level with the last sacral vertebra is the site of injection for *Caudal*.

(g) A continuous anesthetic effect during labor and delivery can be obtained with *Caudal* and *Epidural.*

(h) *Pudendal* is used to block nerves at the ischial spine level to provide anesthesia to the perineal area, vulva, and vagina.

(i) A headache is a side effect of *Spinal* and *Saddle.*

(j) The major side effect of maternal hypotension is associated with *Spinal, Saddle, Caudal,* and *Epidural.*

(k) The *Paracervical* is effective only during Stage I of labor.

(l) The *Saddle* provides anesthesia to the perineum, lower pelvis, and upper thighs.

(m) *Epidural* anesthesia is administered into the space surrounding the dura between L2-L3 or L3-L4.

CHAPTER 8

PREPARED CHILDBIRTH

Patricia D. Williams

Prepared childbirth has gained recognition and acceptance in the United States in the last two decades. In the 1980s, options for a single parent or a couple are numerous, ranging from reading books to attending support group classes. Through childbirth education, the mother and her primary support person can be psychologically and physiologically prepared for the birth experience. Six methods that have influenced the development of prepared childbirth programs are discussed in this chapter, with the Lamaze method being explored in the most depth.

OBJECTIVES

Upon completion of this chapter, the reader will be able to:

1. Compare the reactions of prepared and unprepared women during labor.
2. State three advantages of childbirth preparation.
3. Compare the Read, Bradley, hypnosis, Lamaze, psychosexual (Kitzinger), and New Childbirth (Wright) methods of child-birth preparation.
4. State three benefits of learning and using controlled relaxation techniques.
5. Identify five signs that indicate tension or loss of control during labor and interventions that might alleviate them.

continued on next page

---

6. List, describe, and practice Lamaze breathing patterns that may be used in labor.
7. Identify three techniques used by the support person to assist the mother with relaxation and breathing techniques during labor.
8. Assess a labor situation and formulate a care plan to assist the mother or couple throughout the labor experience.

OVERVIEW OF PREPARED CHILDBIRTH

Reactions to Labor

Through the years, women have been conditioned to fear labor by being told that they might scream and lose control and that labor pains hurt but are forgotten once the baby is born. The word *pain* has been emphasized. Therefore, an unprepared woman may react to the beginning of labor by becoming panicky and fearful. As contractions continue and become more intense, a woman may become uncooperative; she may be unable to concentrate; and she may find herself thinking only about the pain. Tension is evident. She may arch her back, grab hold of the side-rails, and moan or hold her breath. Her inability to relax and breathe regularly contributes to her discomfort during labor. (There is further discussion of pain and reaction to labor in Chapters 1 and 7.)

Relaxation and Breathing During Labor

Effective relaxation and controlled breathing are not instinctive responses to labor contractions but have to be learned and practiced before labor begins. Relaxation techniques and breathing patterns are integral components of each childbirth preparation method. These activities during childbirth provide a point of concentration for the mother and aid in maintaining her comfort and control and in increasing her threshold to pain.

Relaxation may be an active or passive process. Breathing patterns vary and are unique to the specific method being taught. Chest or abdominal muscles are used. The specific patterns are learned and practiced during pregnancy and used during labor and delivery. The key to controlled breathing is controlled relaxation.

Advantages of Preparation for Childbirth

Fear of childbirth is decreased when the expectant mother or couple learn about the physiologic process of childbirth and have the opportunity to discuss fears and concerns with other pregnant women or couples. Childbirth preparation classes are usually conducted by individuals trained in a specific method. Classes are organized to include presentation of factual content about the process of pregnancy and childbirth and practice time and group discussion. In a group situation (as compared with a person learning independently), the group functions as a support system for its members. Parents are encouraged to discuss their feelings and goals with one another and to communicate their concerns and goals to the health care team.

Psychologic and physiologic preparation for childbirth contributes to a positive self-image and the development of coping skills and provides an opportunity for parents to work towards a common goal of a positive birth experience. In addition, the right of the mother or couple to participate actively in the birth of the baby is a demand of many expectant women or couples today.

Review Questions

1. The unprepared mother may react to labor by becoming _____
    ____ , _____ , and _____ .

2. State three reasons why relaxation during labor is important.
    a. _____
    b. _____
    c. _____

3. List three advantages of childbirth preparation.
    a. _____
    b. _____
    c. _____

Answers

1. The unprepared mother may react to labor by becoming panicky, fearful, uncooperative, unable to concentrate, pain oriented in thoughts, and tense.

2. Relaxation during labor is important because it:
    a. provides a point of concentration for the mother.

b. promotes the mother's physical comfort.
c. facilitates the mother's self-control.
d. increases the mother's pain threshold.
3. Advantages of childbirth preparation are:
    a. decreased fear through education about the physical and psychologic process of childbirth.
    b. increased self-confidence in the mother.
    c. development of coping skills in the mother or couple.
    d. active participation of the mother or couple in the birth experience.

METHODS OF CHILDBIRTH PREPARATION

Read Method

In the 1930s, British physician Grantly Dick-Read stressed that labor and delivery is a natural process and called his method of prepared childbirth *natural childbirth*. He theorized that the pain of childbirth is a result of the woman's response of fear and tension to this physiologic process. He referred to this as the Fear-Tension-Pain Syndrome.[1] Thus, education regarding the physiologic process of pregnancy and childbirth as well as specific breathing and passive relaxation techniques would eliminate the fear, reduce the tension, and minimize the pain.

Read's relaxation concept involves relaxation of the mind and progressive relaxation of muscles. This passive relaxation is used both during and between uterine contractions. Emphasis is placed on total body relaxation rather than on conscious relaxation of the tense voluntary muscles.

Abdominal breathing during uterine contractions is taught. By elevating tense abdominal muscles away from the contracting uterus there is less pressure on the sensitive uterus during the contractions.

Although Read did not stress involvement of the husband in the actual event, abdominal breathing and passive relaxation techniques are taught to both parents in preparation for the childbirth experience. Read's method of natural childbirth became known in the United States in the 1960s primarily through one of his books *Childbirth Without Fear,* published in 1944.

Bradley Method

In the 1960s, Robert Bradley, M.D., also promoted a total body relaxation concept of natural childbirth, without the use of medication. He involved the husband in the preparation period as well as in the labor and delivery process. Labor was coached by the husband. His book *Husband Coached Childbirth* includes chapters specifically directed toward the husband (living with a pregnant wife, training rules, role in breastfeeding). Classes in the Bradley method include muscle toning exercises and techniques (perineal exercises, pelvic rock, thigh limbering, nipple preparation), passive relaxation techniques, abdominal breathing patterns, and information about nutrition and environmental variables that affect the pregnancy and birth experience.

To promote deep-relaxation the Bradley method encourages the mother to assume a comfortable resting position, close her eyes, and concentrate on positive thoughts unrelated to the birth experience. She is taught to let her breathing rate flow with the natural body rhythms and responses to labor. This technique enables the woman to disassociate herself from the uterine contractions. The use of abdominal breathing decreases the perception of pain as the abdominal muscles rise up and away from the uterus during inhalation; the depth of breathing remains constant and the release is done slowly yet rhythmically during the exhalation.

The Bradley method emphasizes a family's need for nonseparation following the birth of the baby. In the 1970s, Dr. Bradley continued to expand his philosophy to include focus on a diet that omits foods containing preservatives, added salts, sugars, and animal fats. He further relates human childbirth experiences to those of animals and focuses on the environment, namely decreased noise and light, as a means of making childbirth a more natural experience.

Hypnosis

Hypnotic suggestion as a method of self-help during labor and delivery is not new, having been used in the 1800s and reconsidered in the written work of Chertok in the 1960s. It involves responding to a learned post-hypnotic suggestion.

A hypnotist must first explore the mother's motivation for desiring hypnosis during childbirth. Learning this method may take several months, as the mother must first master the suggestions that enable her to reach a trancelike state while remaining awake, totally relaxed, and responsive to the hypnotist. The extent to which hypnosis can be effective may vary according to the individual's susceptibility and ability to maintain the trancelike state and her ability to respond during labor. The physiologic process of childbirth is discussed. Relaxed breathing patterns are to be used during the course of labor. The time involved and the fact that the hypnotist replaces the supportive role of the father are major reasons why this method is not widely used in the United States.

Review Question

Compare the elements of support person involvement, relaxation techniques, and breathing patterns discussed in the identified childbirth preparation methods.

	Support Person Involvement	Relaxation	Breathing
1. Read:			
2. Bradley:			
3. Hypnosis:			

Answer

1. The Read method advocates natural childbirth with support person involvement during pregnancy, and passive relaxation and abdominal breathing during labor.

2. The Bradley method advocates husband coached childbirth, passive relaxation, and abdominal breathing.

3. The hypnosis method advocates passive relaxation with the hypnotist as the support person and relaxed breathing techniques.

Lamaze Method

Fernand Lamaze, a French obstetrician, developed his theory of conditioned response for childbirth based on the Pavlovian concepts practiced in Russia in the 1930s. He and his monitrice taught the physiologic process of childbirth, proper body mechanics during pregnancy, and comfort measures for pregnancy and labor, along with active relaxation and chest breathing techniques for labor and birth.

The method developed through the years and became widely recognized in the United States in the 1960s through the efforts of Marjorie Karmel, an American woman who had lived in Paris and trained in the method, and who had personally used the method in France. She wrote of her birth experience in the book *Thank You, Dr. Lamaze* in 1959. Other pioneers who established the Lamaze method during the early 1960s were Elizabeth Bing, a physical therapist and childbirth educator, and Irwin Chabon, M.D., an obstetrician from New York, who wrote *Awake* and *Aware* and promoted the philosophy of family-centered maternity care. Two organizations that were established to promote the Lamaze method were the American Society for Psychoprophylaxis in Obstetrics (ASPO), founded in 1961 by a group of obstetricians in New York; and the Childbirth Without Pain Association of Detroit (CWPA), founded by Flora Hummel, R.N., who was trained by Dr. Lamaze and who promoted painless childbirth.[2]

The Lamaze method was originally called painless childbirth, and still is in France. This term met with antagonism from the American medical community, as new medications and regional anesthesia techniques were being developed and widely used to reduce maternal discomfort in labor and delivery. Thus, the term psychoprophylaxis began to be used. This put more emphasis on the effect of the psyche during the labor and birth experience.

The Lamaze method also includes physical preparation through exercises and breathing patterns and relaxation techniques for pregnancy and labor and delivery. Active relaxation is an integral part of the Lamaze method. This is a process whereby the mother concentrates on a focal point, recognizes muscle tension, and works towards achievement of total relaxation of tense voluntary muscles during and between contractions. Since the breathing techniques use the chest muscles, the diaphragm moves up and away from the contracting uterus so that the uterus can expand more effectively.

The breathing patterns may vary according to the intensity of the contractions and the progress of labor. Techniques that can be used during the expulsion phase are also taught. It is felt that the conditioning exercises as well as the use of relaxation and breathing techniques facilitate a more comfortable postpartum recovery phase.[3]

In Lamaze preparation the mother's choice of a support person is most essential. The mother and support person, usually the father, work together during practice sessions at home and in class. This team effort contributes to the development of self-confidence, coping skills, and shared goals for childbirth and parenting.[4]

Psychosexual Method (Kitzinger)

The psychosexual approach was developed in England by Sheila Kitzinger. Using concepts of the Read method, Kitzinger developed a program that included (1) the psychologic and physiologic elements of pain and childbirth; (2) the sensory-memory approach to active relaxation and its use in adapting to the sensations felt and responses that facilitate a flowing with, rather than against, the labor; and (3) the psychosexual aspects of pregnancy and labor and delivery and the postpartum period as one part of the life cycle.

The mother is taught to identify tension and relaxation of muscles during both normal and stressful activities. She is taught to feel the relationship between the muscles of the mouth and the pelvic floor during tension and relaxation through a series of contraction and relaxation exercises. This assists her to understand the role these muscles play in sexual activity and childbirth. Through the use of imagery and touching, she is taught how to consciously relax. Massage and stroking of the back, abdomen, thighs, and perineum by the support person promote relaxation and the feeling of closeness between mother and support person.

Breathing techniques begin with deep, slow breathing and abdominal muscle relaxation, progressing to a deeper chest-accordion type breathing. An upper chest pattern or a mouth breathing technique can be used toward the end of labor. This pattern plus relaxation of the muscles of the pelvic floor facilitates the birth of the baby.

Because Kitzinger feels that the childbearing cycle is a "normal life crisis," she emphasizes the importance of the husband's participation in the total process.[5] Her program addresses the recovery phase following childbirth, including the emotional changes and role adjustment of parents.

The New Childbirth (Wright Method)

The New Childbirth is a term applied to one European approach developed by Erna Wright and the National Childbirth Trust in England. This approach encompasses the principles and some techniques of psychoprophylaxis and is presented in a 1966 text *The New Childbirth*.

Wright focuses on learning relaxation through a series of neuromuscular disassociation drills. The chest breathing patterns differ from other methods in the way they are presented. The patterns are referred to as levels A,B,C,D, which change according to the frequency and intensity of the contraction and allow the woman to switch gears as the contractions accelerate and decelerate. Level A is deep, slow, rhythmic breathing, about 6 cycles per 30 seconds. Level B is a lighter, rhythmic pattern, about 11 cycles per 30 seconds. Level C is a shallow, rhythmic chest breathing, about 35 cycles per 30 seconds. Level D is a chest panting pattern done through an open mouth. A pant-blow breathing pattern, which can be used in transition phases, and breathing for use in the expulsion phase are also taught. The mother can use each level separately or in combination; for example, levels A,B,C,A in one contraction versus only level A in another.[6]

The text in which this method is presented discusses the physiologic and psychologic aspects of pregnancy and childbirth and facilitates learning by the mother and her support person as a couple alone or in a group.

Other Childbirth Preparation Methods

In addition to the methods discussed in this chapter, there are *eclectic* approaches to childbirth preparation. They combine various elements of several methods; for example, the breathing patterns of one method with the relaxation concepts of another. The reader is referred to Sasmor's text, *Childbirth Education: A Nursing Perspective* for further discussion of the eclectic approaches.

The LeBoyer method, which focuses on the effect of birth on the infant, is described in Chapter 9, since it does not involve actual childbirth preparation methods.

Review Question

Compare the elements of support person involvement, relaxation techniques, and breathing patterns discussed in the identified childbirth preparation methods.

	Support Person Involvement	Relaxation	Breathing
1. Lamaze:			
2. Psychosexual (Kitzinger):			
3. New Childbirth (Wright):			

Answer

1. The Lamaze method advocates active support person involvement, active relaxation techniques, and chest breathing patterns.

2.. The Psychosexual (Kitzinger) approach advocates active involvement of the major support person (the husband), the sensory-memory approach to relaxation with focus on touch and stroking, and chest breathing patterns.

3. The New Childbirth (Wright) approach advocates active involvement of a primary-support person, active relaxation, and a breathing approach that combines chest breathing patterns, for example, levels A,B, and/or C, providing for a switching of gears, according to intensity of contractions.

LAMAZE CHILDBIRTH PREPARATION

The Purpose of Psychoprophylactic Childbirth Preparation

In Lamaze childbirth preparation, the mother learns and practices muscle toning exercises, active relaxation and breathing patterns to gain body awareness, and ability to handle the emotional and physical aspects of pregnancy and the efforts of labor. Repeated practice teaches her to actively concentrate and conditions her mind and body to associate uterine contractions of labor with the active relaxation and learned breathing techniques. The process of conditioning increases her pain threshold, thus making labor less painful (not painless, which was an original goal of Lamaze).

Neuromuscular Control

Neuromuscular control, or controlled relaxation, can be defined as "concentration upon active, consciously directed release of voluntary muscles."[7] Benefits of controlled relaxation techniques are numerous. The release of voluntary muscles in labor improves circulation thus increasing oxygenation flow to the uterus and removal of waste products. (Accumulation of waste products in the muscles can cause pain.) The woman is more relaxed and experiences less fatigue and is better able to cope with the efforts of labor. The practice and use of the relaxation techniques provide a framework in which the couple can learn to work together. In labor, the uterine contraction is the painful stimulus. The body's response may be one of tension or a conditioned response of controlled relaxation and breathing techniques. For more information about the neurologic responses to pain and the conditioned response of controlled relaxation, the reader is referred to Hassid's text, *Textbook for Childbirth Educators*.

Review Question

State three purposes of psychoprophylactic childbirth preparation.

1. _____

2. _____

3. _____

Answer

Purposes of psychoprophylactic childbirth preparation are:
1. to gain body awareness and ability to handle effects of labor.

2. to increase ability to concentrate and condition the body to associate contractions with active relaxation and breathing techniques.

3. to teach techniques that decrease physical and mental discomfort.

Positioning

Comfortable positioning is a prerequisite to relaxation. A position of comfort should be assumed during practice sessions as well as during the actual birth process. The following points should be followed for comfortable positioning. The back should be supported with a pillow, rolled towel, or warm water bottle underneath or behind the lumbar portion. The arms should be supported. When in a sitting position, the feet may rest on a foot stool; when extended, the legs may rest directly on the floor or may be supported with pillows under the knees and/or heels. Flexibility is a key element in the support process. The mother does not always know which will be the most comfortable laboring position. Thus, she is encouraged to try various positions, many of which are discussed in Chapters 3 and 9.

Concentration

Concentration is a part of the relaxation (neuromuscular control) process. The ability to concentrate improves with practice. Concentration is enhanced by the use of a focal point (an object or specific area to look at which is stationary, easily recognized, and consistent). A mother may bring her focal point into a labor room or select a specific point (avoiding the clock) in the room to concentrate on during each contraction. This is an active process, not passive and sleep inducing, and acts as a diversionary technique from the pain of the contraction. Once the mother is comfortable and has a focal point, she can concentrate on relaxing all the voluntary muscles of her body during the contraction. This is an effective psychologic and a positive physical response to the contraction.

Breathing

When concentrating, a woman sometimes has a tendency to hold her breath. She should learn to breathe comfortably using mouth and nasal breathing. As she practices relaxation exercises she should take a *relaxing breath* (deep breath in through the nose and out through the mouth) at the beginning and end of each exercise. This will aid in conditioning her to respond to activity in labor by beginning and ending each contraction with a relaxing breath (cleansing breath).

Recognizing Tension

The mother must learn to recognize tension prior to practicing relaxation techniques. To be of assistance to the laboring woman, the support person must also recognize tension and can do so by practicing exercises that consist of the elements of concentration, muscle tension, and conscious, active relaxation. When learning neuromuscular control it is important to become aware of the body's muscles, to feel what it is like to tense them, and then to feel what it is like to relax them.

A comfortable position must be assumed for practice. In the beginning, it is best to select a sitting or semi-sitting position in a comfortable chair. If lying on the floor, pillows should be used to support legs (side-lying) or to elevate the head and shoulders. When one is in a sitting position, feet can be supported on a stool or the floor.

The following exercise focuses on identification of tension and corresponding relaxation. It is a combination of several specific tension/release exercises. Instructions should be followed carefully.

EXERCISE: TENSION AND RELEASE (for practice)
Assume your comfortable position.
Take a relaxing breath; find your focal point.
Tense your forehead by frowning; slowly relax your forehead to the count of ten.
Tense your mouth by putting the tip of the tongue on the roof of the mouth; slowly relax your tongue to the count of ten.
Tense your lower jaw (clinch teeth together); slowly relax your jaw to the count of ten.
Tense your right arm and hand while totally relaxing all other muscles in your body; slowly relax your right arm and hand.
Proceed in the same manner with your left arm and hand.
Tense your upper back by arching your back; slowly relax your upper back to the count of ten.
Tense your lower back by pressing against the back of the chair or floor; slowly relax your lower back to the count of ten.
Tense your right leg and foot while totally relaxing all other muscles in your body. Slowly relax your right leg and foot.

Proceed in the same manner with your left leg and foot.
Take a slow, relaxing breath. Relax completely.

As you worked through this exercise you may have felt tension in several parts of your body, thus finding it difficult to voluntarily relax your muscles. The woman in labor can experience the same difficulties. The problem is usually related to concentration, breathing, or body position. The areas of tension, the objective signs, and suggested interventions are summarized in the following chart.

AREAS OF TENSION	OBJECTIVE SIGNS	INTERVENTIONS
A. Face/Neck	a. Grimace, frown, scowl.	Relax face. Have eye contact with support person.
	b. Moaning, gritting of teeth.	Relax face and mouth.
	c. Breath-holding.	Take a relaxing breath.
		Concentrate on focal point.
		Receive words of encouragement.
B. Arms/Hands	a. Clutching pillow, siderails and coach's hand.	Rest arms on bed or pillow.
	b. Shoulders firm to touch.	Rest hands on lap, bed.
		Change positions.
C. Back	a. Back firm to touch.	Have back stroked by coach.
	b. Arching back.	Place pillow, rolled towel, warm water bottle against back.
D. Legs/Feet	a. Toes stiff, feet tense.	Support legs, put pillows under knees, feet.
	b. Legs stretched out.	Have thighs, legs stroked.

The tension and release exercises will help increase awareness of tension and active relaxation in complex muscle groups. These exercises are for practice only, not for use in labor. Relaxation, not tension, is the focus for labor.

Recognizing Relaxation

The identification of and practicing of controlled relaxation prior to labor make it easier to relax during actual labor. Although mothers who have not had childbirth preparation may find it very difficult to concentrate and relax, they can try to participate actively. Thus, the availability of a knowledgeable nurse or support person is of great benefit to the unprepared mother.

The following exercise focuses totally on the relaxation process as an active relaxation of the voluntary muscles. It can also be used in early labor prior to use of specific breathing patterns.

EXERCISE: CONCENTRATION AND RELAXATION
Assume your comfortable position.
Take a relaxing breath; find your focal point.
Relax your face and neck completely.
Relax your arms and hands.
Relax your chest, then your abdomen.
Relax your back, then your buttocks.
Relax your legs and feet.
Take a slow, relaxing breath. Now your body should be completely relaxed.

It is most efficient to learn by separating the exercises into muscle groups such as the arms and legs, face and neck, chest, abdomen, and back. The learning of these exercises should take place over a period of several weeks. During the last few weeks of pregnancy, a mother is encouraged to practice each day by herself and with her support person. In general, long sessions each day yield no more pain relief in labor than short daily sessions of five or ten minutes each. Thus the regularity of practice is more important than infrequent, long practice sessions.[8]

Review Questions

1. List five signs of tension that may be exhibited by the woman in labor.
   a. _____
   b. _____
   c. _____
   d. _____
   e. _____

2. A relaxing breath is taken _____ of each contraction.

Answers

1. The woman in labor may indicate tension by
   a. grimacing, frowning, scowling.
   b. moaning, gritting teeth.
   c. breath-holding.
   d. clutching the pillow, siderails, coach's hand.
   e. tightening the shoulders and back muscles.
   f. arching the back.
   g. stretching legs and stiffening the toes.

2. A relaxing breath is taken *at the beginning and end* of each contraction.

Activities Promoting Relaxation in Labor

Labor contractions can be intense and, for some women, more painful than expected. The constant presence of and communication with the support person are her main sources of reassurance. Generally, a woman in labor does not wish to be alone. Should the support person temporarily leave, it is important that the mother be told and a nurse or a friend assume that role.

If the mother has difficulty or if she has had no previous preparation, the support person may actually have to show her how to relax. This can be done by touching the muscles and telling her if she is relaxed. *Effleurage* or stroking, which is a gentle massaging of the skin, assists in relaxing tense muscles.

Supporting activities that promote relaxation in labor may be time consuming for the coach. A woman in labor responds best to a support person who is relaxed. If the support person has practiced the exercises previously discussed, he or she has felt muscle tension and is aware of the purposes of active relaxation techniques in labor.

Purpose of Regulated Breathing Patterns in Labor

Specific breathing as well as relaxation patterns are conditioned responses used to cope with labor. In the normal breathing cycle, expansion of the rib cage, intercostal muscles, and lungs occurs upon inhalation. At the same time there is downward movement of the diaphragm towards the uterus. The same muscles and structures move upward toward the lungs upon exhalation. Specific regulated chest breathing patterns facilitate the mother's comfort by decreasing diaphragmatic pressure on the contracting uterus and promoting oxygenation in the mother and fetus.

The rate (speed) and the rhythm of the pattern are as important as the muscles used. Studies have shown that the breathing patterns are more effective in increasing the pain threshold when the mother can select the technique and rate to be used during the contraction.[9]

As labor progresses, the body's reaction is tension and a tendency toward uncontrolled breathing. Breathing that is done by using the chest muscles, inhalation through the nose, and exhalation through the mouth may enable the mother to relax and breathe at a regular pace. Breathing techniques promote concentration and foster relaxation.

Relaxing Breath

A relaxing breath (cleansing breath) is taken at the beginning and end of each contraction just as it was before and after each relaxation exercise. The relaxing breath is a complete respiratory cycle of inhaling through the nose deeply and then passively exhaling through the mouth. It gives the mother extra oxygen to work with, helps her concentrate on the specific patterns, and signals the support person that the contraction is beginning or ending. The breath may be up to 10 seconds long and is deeper than in regular breathing. The tip of the tongue may be placed on the roof of the mouth or behind the top of the bottom teeth to decrease the drying of the oral mucosa.

Hyperventilation

Hyperventilation is a problem that may occur during practice of breathing patterns and in labor. It is a state of carbon dioxide deficiency within the body and is produced by irregular breathing and exhaling too deeply or too often. Signs of hyperventilation include dizziness, panic, tingly or numb sensation around the fingers or mouth, and stiff fingers. To correct this state, all or any one of the following may be done by the woman:
1. Blow in and out into a paper bag throughout the contraction until the feelings of hyperventilation diminish.
2. Cup hands over the mouth and breathe into them during the contraction.
3. Hold air in for a few seconds at the end of the contraction and then slowly (not forcefully) release it.

While learning patterns prior to labor, it is relatively easy to hyperventilate, because the patterns are not those of normal breathing. Hyperventilation can occur because the mother is tense or scared. It is important for the support person to recognize signs of hyperventilation in order to assist the mother in coping with this syndrome and regaining control.

Review Questions

Select the correct response(s).

1. During normal inspiration, the diaphragm:
   a. moves downward toward the uterus.
   b. moves upward toward the lungs.

2. Hyperventilation may occur in labor because of:
   a. muscle tension.
   b. inhalation of too much oxygen.
   c. breathing irregularities.
   d. exhaling too deeply.

3. Hyperventilation may be corrected by:
   a. inhaling oxygen from a mask throughout the contraction.
   b. breathing into a paper bag throughout the contraction.
   c. blowing into cupped hands at the end of the contraction.
   d. holding air in the lungs for a few seconds at the end of the contraction.

Answers

1. During inspiration (a) the diaphragm moves downward toward the uterus.

2. Hyperventilation may occur in labor because of:
   a. muscle tension.
   b. inhalation of too much oxygen.
   c. breathing irregularities.
   d. exhaling too deeply.

3. Hyperventilation may be corrected by:
   b. breathing into a paper bag or cupped hands throughout the contraction.
   d. holding air in lungs for a few seconds at the end of the contraction.

Specific Lamaze Breathing Techniques that May Be Used During Labor

In the United States, the specific breathing patterns that a mother may use in labor encompass a variety of rates and rhythms and may vary according to the region in which the Lamaze class is offered.

SLOW CHEST BREATHING. This pattern can be used when relaxation, regular breathing, and comfort measures are no longer effective in controlling the discomforts of labor. Inhalation is done through the nose more deeply than during normal breathing, yet not so deeply that air is forced in and pressure felt on the abdomen or uterus. A relaxed exhalation is done through the mouth.

A suggested pattern follows: with the mouth shut, inhale through the nose for 1 to 2 seconds, open mouth, relax jaw and lips, and slowly release air for 3 to 4 seconds. An approximate rate is 6 to 12 respiratory cycles per minute. Each contraction will begin and end with a relaxing breath. Slow chest breathing is rhythmic and continued throughout the contraction. The use of effleurage with early breathing patterns may facilitate concentration and enhance the effectiveness of the technique.

The pattern is diagrammed as follows:

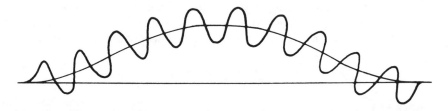

As labor progresses, the slow, rhythmic chest breathing may no longer be effective. The mother may then move on to another chest breathing pattern.

SHALLOW CHEST BREATHING. This is more active, shallow inhalation through the nose for 1 second and exhalation through a relaxed mouth for 1 second. The amount of air inhaled is the same as the amount exhaled. Breathing cycles number about 30 per minute. This pattern is maintained throughout the contraction and is diagrammed as follows:

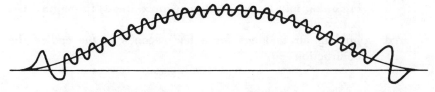

As contractions continue and become more intense, the mother may vary the rate of this pattern and flow with the contraction. Thus, she may begin with the in-1, out-1 rate, accelerate to in-out in 1 second, and then decelerate with the in-1, out-1 pattern. Increasing breathing rate during the peak of the contraction is a normal response.

SHALLOW PANT-BLOW BREATHING. This light shallow pant with a blow is done through the mouth. During the breathing cycle, the tip of the tongue is put on the roof of the mouth (to moisten and filter air as it enters the mouth) or behind the lower teeth. The blow is more forceful and deliberate through pursed lips. This pattern can be used when additional techniques are needed to help the mother cope with labor and also when the urge to push needs to be controlled. Each pant is in and out in one second and the blow is out for two seconds or more. The pattern is determined by the intensity of the contraction; thus, the mother increases the panting rate and blows out more frequently as the contraction or pushing urge becomes more intense. She then slows the panting and blows out less as the contraction decelerates.

The pattern is diagrammed as follows:

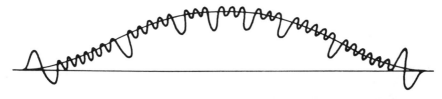

A variation of the pant-blow pattern is the "F" blow, whereby the mother may pronounce the letter "F" on the exhale blow.[10] This may be less strenuous and more effective in controlling an urge to push.

A "puff-blow" pattern may be used in lieu of "pant-blow." The puff-blow is done like the shallow breathing with the addition of a blow. The mother can vary the rhythm with the intensity of the contraction.[11]

SHALLOW CHEST PANTING. If pant-blow breathing is not an effective tool for handling the contractions at this time, and as the mother moves into second stage, continuous, rhythmic chest panting may prove effective. This pattern is done by putting the tip of the tongue on the roof of the mouth and panting in and out through the mouth in a shallow regulated pattern. The mother should take a relaxing-cleansing breath at the beginning and end of the contraction. The rate is steady and is influenced (faster-slower) by the intensity of the contraction.

The pattern is diagrammed as follows:

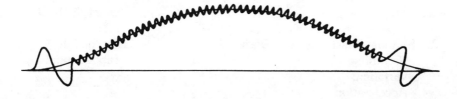

Review Questions

Name the pattern that is described as follows:

1. Slow, rhythmic breathing; 6–12 cycles per minute; effleurage may be helpful at this time. _____
2. Active, shallow breathing; approximately 30 cycles per minute. _____
3. Light, shallow pant with a blow; pattern determined by intensity of the contraction and pushing urge. _____
4. Light, rhythmic panting pattern; may be used as mother moves into 2nd stage. _____

Answer

1. Slow Chest Breathing

2. Shallow Chest Breathing

3. Shallow Pant-Blow Breathing

4. Shallow Chest Panting Breathing

Several breathing patterns have been discussed. The patterns, difficulties that may be encountered, and interventions for coping with the difficulties are summarized in the following chart.

BREATHING PATTERNS	PROBLEM	INTERVENTION
1. Slow Chest Breathing	a. Lack of air	a. Take a deeper relaxing breath.
		b. Increase the pace a little.
		c. Regulate the count: in 2-out 2,3,4".
2. Shallow Chest Breathing Variation: Acceleration/ Deceleration	a. Dizzy	a. Breathe into cupped hands.

3. Shallow Pant-Blow Breathing Variations: "F Blow"/"Puff-Blow"	a. Tingly	a. Take a relaxing breath.
		b. Breathe at a regular pace.
		c. Keep breathing shallow and high in the chest.
		d. Change to a more comfortable position.
4. Shallow Chest Panting	a. Fatigue	a. Slow the breathing rate.
	b. Hyperventilation	b. Focus on focal point.
		c. Breathe into cupped hands.
		d. Breathe in and out into a paper bag.
		e. Hold breath at end of the contraction (for a few seconds) until feeling passes and exhalation is needed.

Depending on the physical and emotional well being of the mother and the position of the infant, a variety of comfort positions may be used along with the breathing patterns as the mother progresses through the first stage of labor. Breathing toward the end of this first stage may be dependent on the need to push and include the pant-blow or panting technique previously discussed. Guidelines for pushing as well as positioning for pushing are discussed in Chapter 9.

Activities Supporting Breathing Patterns in Labor

The support person is encouraged to practice the breathing patterns to gain an awareness of the techniques and the problems that a woman in labor may have to cope with. Activities such as timing the contractions, recognizing when the mother is having difficulty with breathing patterns, and helping her with changes in techniques are of great assistance to both prepared and unprepared mothers.

Timing and pacing contractions are essential when assisting the mother with the breathing patterns. Pacing can be defined as the verbal coaching of the woman through the contraction by the use of verbal cues such as "contraction begins," "15 seconds, 30 seconds" or "half over, almost over," "contraction ends." When timing contractions, the support person can time from the beginning of one contraction until the beginning of the next. This time period includes the contraction and the rest period. These cues offered by the support person help the mother work more effectively through the contractions.[12]

Verbal and nonverbal clues that the woman in labor gives her support person might indicate that she is losing control and that she desires to switch to another breathing pattern. It is important that the support person be aware of these signs, as the fear of losing control can be a frightening fear during labor. The following clues may indicate loss of control: tension and restlessness by scowling, gritting the teeth, holding the support person's hand, or arching the back; moaning or saying "It hurts more;" omission of the relaxing breath; and difficulty with the breathing pattern and relaxation response.

The prepared mother is conditioned to respond to the contraction with positive activities such as breathing, relaxing, and responding to her support person's commands. Words such as "relax," "slow down," "speed up," and "It's almost over," are common commands which the support person may use. The prepared mother who practices the relaxation and breathing combinations independently can handle some contractions herself.

When working with the unprepared mother, the nurse can explain in simple language and demonstrate pacing and timing contractions using her or his own commands. Because this mother is not conditioned to respond immediately to breathing and relaxation commands, adaptation to the techniques is altered. However, this mother can be assisted to work with her contractions and actively participate in her childbirth experience.

An important function of the support person is to recognize the need for breathing pattern changes, to coach the mother's breathing throughout the contraction, and if needed, to breathe with her to get her started into the pattern. The support person is concerned about the rate and rhythm of the pattern as well as the concentrated effort of the mother. One difficulty the mother may have when doing regulated breathing patterns is that of a dry, bad-tasting mouth. Aides such as ice chips, lollipops, a cold cloth to suck on, and glycerine swabs are refreshing and make the mouth taste better; thus, breathing is easier and more relaxing.

The support person also helps the mother maintain a comfortable position to help cope with contractions. It is difficult to relax and breathe comfortably during labor. (See Chapters 3 and 9 and the relaxation portion of this chapter.) For this reason the support person should help the woman in labor change positions periodically throughout her labor. The prepared couple has often worked out comfortable ways of practicing techniques and the commands to be used during the contractions. The mother learns to respond to her support person's voice. The support person is an essential element of the Lamaze method.

Review Question

1. List three measures that may be used in coaching breathing techniques.
   a. _____
   b. _____
   c. _____

Answer

1. The coach assists during labor by:
   a. timing, pacing, and determining contraction patterns.
   b. breathing with the mother.
   c. offering the mother ice chips and a cold cloth to suck on.
   d. reminding the mother to relax, breathe, and concentrate on the focal point.

REFERENCES

1. DICK-READ, G: *Childbirth Without Fear,* ed 2. Harper & Row, New York, 1959.
2. HASSID, P: *Textbook For Childbirth Educators.* Harper & Row, Hagerstown, 1978, p 174.
3. HASSID, P: *Textbook for Childbirth Educators.* Harper & Row, Hagerstown, 1978, pp 29,32.
4. JIMENEZ, SL: *Education for the childbearing year: Comprehensive application of psychoprophylaxis.* J Obstet Gynecol Neonatal Nurs 9(2):97, 1980.
5. KITZINGER, S: *The Experience of Childbirth.* Penguin Books, Baltimore, 1967.
6. WRIGHT, E: *The New Childbirth.* Hart Publishing, New York, 1966.
7. HASSID, P: *Textbook for Childbirth Educators.* Harper & Row, Hagerstown, 1978, p 176.

8. COGAN, R: *Practice time in prepared childbirth.* J Obstet Gynecol Neonatal Nurs 7(1):33, 1978.
9. WORTHINGTON, EL, ET AL: *Which prepared childbirth coping strategies are effective?* J Obstet Gynecol Neonatal Nurs 11(1):45, 1982, p 51.
10. *Lamaze Childbirth and Parenting Handbook,* ed 2. Ann Arbor, 1978, p 42.
11. HASSID, P: *Textbook for Childbirth Educators.* Harper & Row, Hagerstown, 1978, p 185.
12. WORTHINGTON, EL, ET AL: *Which prepared childbirth coping strategies are effective?* J Obstet Gynecol Neonatal Nurs 11(1):45; 1982. p 51.

BIBLIOGRAPHY

BRADLEY, R: *Husband-Coached Childbirth.* Harper & Row, New York, 1974.

CHABON, I: *Awake and Aware.* Dell Publishing, New York, 1966.

COGAN, R: *Practice time in prepared childbirth.* J Obstet Gynecol Neonatal Nurs 7:1:33 1978.

DICK-READ, G: *Childbirth Without Fear,* ed 2. Harper & Row, New York, 1959.

EWY, D AND EWY, R: *A Lamaze Guide: Preparation for Childbirth.* New American Library, New York, 1972.

GENEST, M: *Preparation for childbirth—Evidence for efficacy: A review.* J Obstet Gynecol Neonatal Nurs 10(2):82, 1981.

HASSID, P: *Textbook for Childbirth Educators.* Harper & Row, Hagerstown, 1978.

JIMENEZ, S: *Education for the childbearing year: Comprehensive application of psychoprophylaxis.* J Obstet Gynecol Neonatal Nurs 9(2):97, 1980.

JOHNSON, JM: *Teaching self-hypnosis in pregnancy, labor, and delivery.* Am J Maternal Child Nurs 5(2):99, 1980.

KITZINGER, S: *The Experience of Childbirth.* Penguin Books, Baltimore, 1967.

LAMAZE, F: *Painless Childbirth.* Pocket Books, New York, 1972.

L.C.P.A. *Childbirth and Parenting Handbook,* ed 2. (1978) Lamaze Childbirth Preparation Association of Ann Arbor, Inc., P.O. Box 1816, Ann Arbor, Mi. 48106.

Maternity Center Association: *A Baby is Born.* Grosset and Dunlap, New York, 1964.

McKAY, S: *Maternal position during labor and birth: A reassessment.* J Obstet Gynecol Neonatal Nurs 9(5):288, 1980.

OLDS, S, ET AL: *Obstetric Nursing.* Addison-Wesley, Menlo Park Calif, 1980.

SASMOR, J: *Childbirth Education: A Nursing Perspective.* John Wiley & Sons, New York, 1976.

WRIGHT, E: *The New Childbirth.* Hart Publishing, New York, 1966.

WORTHINGTON, E, MARTIN, G, AND SHUMATE, M: *Which prepared childbirth coping strategies are effective?* J Obstet Gynecol Neonatal Nurs 11(1):45, 1982.

POST TEST

1. Complete the following chart comparing the reactions of the prepared and unprepared mother to labor.

	Prepared	Unprepared
a. Cooperation		
b. Tension		
c. Breathing		
d. Concentration		
e. Emotional State		

2. State three advantages of childbirth preparation.

   a. _____

   b. _____

   c. _____

3. Select the additional corresponding numbers that describe concepts and techniques learned in the following methods of childbirth preparation.

a.	Read	2, _____	1.	Active relaxation
b.	Bradley	2, _____	2.	Passive relaxation
c.	Hypnosis	2, _____	3.	Chest breathing
d.	Lamaze	2, _____	4.	Abdominal breathing
e.	Psychosexual (Kitzinger)	1, _____	5.	Husband-coached childbirth
f.	New Childbirth (Wright)	1, _____	6.	Natural childbirth
			7.	Psychoprophylaxis
			8.	Trancelike state
			9.	Physiologic process of childbirth
			10.	Emotional aspects of childbearing
			11.	Psychosexual approach
			12.	Levels of breathing (gear shifting)

4. State three benefits of controlled relaxation techniques.
   a. _____
   b. _____
   c. _____

5. List five signs that indicate tension or loss of control and the corresponding interventions that assist the mother to regain control.

Signs	Interventions
a. _____	_____
b. _____	_____
c. _____	_____
d. _____	_____
e. _____	

6. Describe the following Lamaze breathing patterns and their rate and use in labor.
   a. Slow Chest Breathing: _____

   b. Shallow Chest Breathing: _____

   c. Shallow Pant-Blow Breathing: _____

   d. Shallow Chest Panting: _____

7. Describe three techniques used by the support person in assisting the woman in labor with relaxation and breathing patterns.
   a. _____
   b. _____
   c. _____

8. Mrs. A. attended Lamaze childbirth preparation classes. She is 4 cm. dilated when you arrive and is doing slow chest breathing. She is complaining of a backache. Contractions are regular, every 4 minutes, lasting 50–60 seconds. After using the slow chest breathing pattern for two more hours, Mrs. A. states that she "feels like she isn't getting enough air" and that "It hurts more now." She begins scowling and moaning during the contractions.

Formulate a coaching plan for Mrs. A. State at least three needs, corresponding supportive measures, and the rationale for each.

Mrs. A's Need	Supportive Measure	Rationale

ANSWERS

1. Reactions of the prepared and unprepared mother to labor are compared in the following chart:

	Prepared	Unprepared
a. Cooperation	Tries to cooperate	Has difficulty cooperating
b. Tension	Practices muscle release	Becomes very tense
c. Breathing	Uses regulated breathing patterns	Breathes fast, irregularly, holds breath
d. Concentration	Has a focal point Concentrates well	Concentrates on pain
e. Emotional state	Is controlled Participates	Is panicky, fearful

2. Advantages of childbirth preparation methods are:
   a. Physical preparation for the childbearing process.
   b. Increased self-confidence.
   c. Development of coping skills.
   d. Opportunity for parents to work towards a common goal.
3. Concepts that describe the following childbirth preparation approaches are:
   a. Read: 2,4,6,9
   b. Bradley: 2,4,5,6,9
   c. Hypnosis: 2,8,9

d. Lamaze:1,3,5,7,9,10
e. Psychosexual (Kitzinger): 1,3,5,6,9,10,11
f. New Childbirth (Wright): 1,3,5,7,9,10,12

4. Benefits of controlled relaxation techniques are:
a. improved circulation during labor, which increases oxygenation for mother and fetus.
b. less fatigue for the mother, thus increasing her ability to work through the contractions.
c. provision of a framework for the couple to work together.

5. Signs of tension or loss of control and support person interventions are:
a. Facial grimace, frown: use words of encouragement to relax facial muscles.
b. Clutching pillow, arching back: support extremities with pillows, assist mother with change of position, massage tense muscles.
c. Breath-holding; other breathing difficulties: breathe with mother and pace contractions.
d. Hyperventilation: assist mother to breathe into cupped hands or hold air in at contraction's end.
e. Moaning, verbalizing: remind to relax, stroke, massage, switch breathing patterns.

6. The primary Lamaze breathing patterns are differentiated as follows:
a. *Slow Chest Breathing:* use of intercostal muscles, breathing in through the nose and out through the mouth; suggested rate of in 1-2, out-3-4, 6–12 respiratory cycles per minute; used when relaxation techniques and basic comfort measures no longer help.
b. *Shallow Chest Breathing:* more active, shallow inhalation through the nose for 1 second and exhalation through the mouth; suggested rate of in-1, out-1, 30 cycles per minute; used when rhythmic chest breathing is no longer effective.
c. *Shallow Pant-Blow Breathing:* light shallow pant with a blow, in and out through the mouth; pattern determined by intensity of the contraction; used when other techniques not effective and for controlling pushing urge.
d. *Shallow Chest Panting:* rhythmic chest panting, in and out through the mouth; rate influenced by intensity of contraction; used to control the pushing urge, or to assist with the expulsion phase.

7. The support person assists the woman in labor with relaxation and breathing patterns by:
a. assisting her in assuming comfortable positions and with comforting measures such as a back rub, back pressure, and passive pelvic rock.

b.   reminding her of her focal point and concentration efforts.

c.   remaining with her and offering verbal praise, encouragement, and reassurance.

d.   checking her voluntary muscles for tension/relaxation.

e.   explaining what is happening and what he or she (the support person) is doing.

8. *Woman's Need*	*Supporting Measure*	*Rationale*
A. Emotional support	a. Reassure b. Explain what is happening c. Remain with mother d. Praise, encourage	The laboring woman does not want to be left alone. Active labor makes it difficult to think of labor's end.
B. Comfort	a. Assist into a comfortable position b. Apply back pressure/massage/effleurage c. Apply warm or cold compresses d. Offer ice chips	Comfortable position promotes relaxation. Pressure and massage; put counterpressure on the presenting part of fetus.
C. Encouragement	a. Remind to use relaxing breath and to concentrate b. Assist with comfort measures c. Remind to use focal point d. Apply touch relaxation	Release of muscles allows for increased blood supply to the uterus. Relaxation is a technique for concentrating on something other than uterine contractions.
D. Assistance with breathing patterns during contractions.	a. Time, pace conctractions b. Praise; be firm if necessary c. Breathe with her if needed d. Check rate and rhythm of breathing pattern e. Coach pant-blow pattern for pushing urge	A pattern needs to be established to assess need to alter breathing pattern. In transition, women need firmness to respond as the pushing urge can be instinctive.

CHAPTER 9

ALTERNATIVES IN CHILDBIRTH

Joyce Bagrowski McCabe

Today couples who are having children are seeking highly personalized, family-centered births. They desire and have the right to an active role in making decisions about their childbirth experience. As a result, there is growing pressure for health care professionals to develop alternatives to traditional birth settings and routine obstetric practices. Some areas of the country have already adopted innovative programs, and others are undergoing the slow process of change. This chapter introduces the reader to several alternatives available to families. It is divided into Alternative Birth Settings and Alternative Practices during Labor and Birth.

OBJECTIVES

Upon completion of this chapter, the reader will be able to:

1. Identify one traditional and three nontraditional birth settings.
2. Compare the advantages and disadvantages of each setting.
3. Recognize conditions that contraindicate giving birth in a nontraditional setting.
4. List alternatives to common early labor routines.
5. Discuss advantages and disadvantages of having friends or family, including children, present at birth.
6. Provide anticipatory guidance for parents who desire their children's presence at the birth of a new baby.

continued on next page

ALTERNATIVE BIRTH SETTINGS

The Conduct of Birth in Various Settings

The following case studies briefly describe the events surrounding birth in the traditional hospital setting and in the nontraditional settings of a birthing room, an alternative birth center, and a home. Although in reality, every birth is not conducted in the same way in each setting, the situations described represent a typical birth in that particular setting.

Case 1. Upon admission to the *hospital labor room*, Cathy was given a perineal shave and an enema, while Ed waited in the lounge. After admission procedures were completed, Ed joined Cathy in the labor room and began coaching her through contractions. Cathy used the breathing and relaxing techniques that she and Ed had learned in Lamaze classes; she was given Demerol 50 mg when the techniques seemed ineffective. Fluids were given intravenously and her membranes were ruptured artificially so that internal electronic monitoring could be implemented. Cathy remained in bed for the rest of her labor, with Ed standing at her side. Nurses periodically checked the contractions and fetal heart rate on the monitor and provided encouragement. A resident checked her progress vaginally as needed.

Upon complete cervical dilatation, Cathy began to push and was transferred to the delivery room when the fetal head was crowning. Following instructions, Ed waited in the hall as Cathy was placed on the delivery table with legs up in stirrups, and draped with sterile sheets. Ed was then invited in and positioned on a stool at Cathy's head. The nurse set up a mirror so they both could watch the delivery. The doctor gave Cathy a local anesthetic into the perineum, made an episiotomy, and instructed Cathy to push.

After three more contractions, the baby was born. The doctor called out, "It's a boy!" and held the baby up for Cathy and Ed to see. They watched and waited eagerly as the nurse dried the baby, instilled silver nitrate drops in the baby's eyes, and carried out the identification procedures. The nurse then wrapped the baby snuggly and gave him to Ed to hold. After the episiotomy was repaired and Cathy was moved onto a stretcher, the nurse provided Cathy with the opportunity to hold and breastfeed her baby. Shortly thereafter, Cathy was taken to the recovery room, the baby to the nursery, and an ecstatic Ed left the hospital.

Case 2. Sue was admitted to the *birthing room* in active labor. The room, previously a labor room, now had a bright yellow bedspread and curtains, flowered wallpaper, and hanging plants. In order to have access to the birthing room, Sue and Tom attended Lamaze classes as well as an orientation class on preparation for use of the birthing room.

Sue sat in the reclining chair or walked around the room during most of the first stage of her labor. Tom stayed at her side, stroking her arms and legs during the contractions to help her relax. The nurse frequently encouraged Sue to drink apple juice or water. No IV was used. The fetal heart rate was auscultated often; a Doptone was used so the parents could also hear.

Upon complete dilatation, the nurse positioned Sue so she could push while sitting up in bed on a birthing stool. When the fetal head was crowning, the nurse brought delivery supplies out of the cupboard and the doctor placed one sterile sheet under Sue's buttocks. He then gave Sue a local anesthetic and made an episiotomy.

Immediately following the birth, the doctor placed the baby on Sue's bare abdomen. He then clamped the cord, handed Tom the scissors, and showed him where to cut. With the baby still on Sue's abdomen, the nurse dried the baby and covered her with a warm dry blanket. After Sue nursed the baby, the nurse did the initial baby care and then gave her to Tom to hold. Sue and Tom remained together with the baby for over an hour; the nurse periodically assessed Sue's vital signs, fundus, and lochia, and the baby's vital signs. The nurse then took Sue, accompanied by Tom, to her postpartum room and the baby to the nursery.

Case 3. Peggy was admitted to the *alternative birth center* with ruptured membranes and mild contractions. The birth center is located in a remodeled house, five minutes driving time from the hospital. Peggy spent her early labor reading to her two children in the birth center's family room and walking with them in the yard. As her contractions became stronger, Peggy and John quietly went into the bedroom. The children continued playing outside or in the family room under the close supervision of Peggy's mother. They looked in on their parents occasionally but were more interested in watching TV.

Peggy walked about the bedroom during most of her labor, leaning against John for support during contractions. She drank her own herbal tea and played her favorite albums on the center's stereo. The certified nurse-midwife quietly praised and encouraged the couple and frequently assessed the fetal heart rate with a Doptone.

When Peggy was completely dilated, she leaned against John in the double bed and began to gently push. The nurse-midwife set up the delivery supplies and applied warm compresses to Peggy's perineum as the baby's head began to crown. As the uncut perineum stretched around the baby's head, Peggy gently pushed it out at the end of a contraction. After the nurse-midwife eased out the baby's shoulders, Peggy reached down and lifted the baby up onto her bare abdomen. No effort was made to separate the baby from her parents; necessary assessments were made without interference in the attachment process.

Peggy and John spent a quiet twenty minutes with the newest member of their family before calling the children in to see and hold their new sister. They all celebrated by singing "Happy Birthday" and opening presents which the parents had brought for the children. The nurse-midwife unobtrusively checked Peggy's vital signs, fundus, and lochia; an hour later she applied erythromycin ointment in the baby's eyes, and weighed, printed, and thoroughly examined the healthy baby.

The family went home together six hours after the birth. In addition to a refresher Lamaze class, Peggy and John attended two classes to prepare them for the birth center and this early discharge. The nurse-midwife planned to maintain contact with them by phone for the next two days and to visit them in their home on the third postpartum day, unless an earlier visit was warranted.

Case 4. Barb was pleased that her planned *home birth* would soon occur; the family was prepared. Barb had taken her children to her prenatal check-ups, allowed them to hear and feel the baby, and encouraged their questions. Barb and Bob had repeatedly explained pictures of babies being born.

Barb phoned the certified nurse-midwife to notify her of the onset of labor. She also phoned her best friend who would watch the children, and her mother who wanted to be there. Barb and her eight-year-old daughter, Jill, changed the sheets, padded the bed, and gathered the supplies. The nurse-midwife and her RN associate arrived. After determining the adequacy of the physical environment, the nurse-midwife monitored Barb's vital signs and contractions, and the fetal heart rate, and performed a vaginal exam. The nurse-midwife phoned her back-up physician to inform him of the situation. The RN set up the supplies for the birth along with equipment brought to handle complications should they occur (IVs, oxytocin, a small oxygen tank, Ambu bags, and so forth).

Jill remained at her mother's side throughout the labor, while the younger children played outside. Jill was the "gopher"—going for ice, lemonade, and cold wet washcloths. Bob coached Barb to breathe through the contractions, and her mother provided encouragement. The nurse-midwife remained nearby, auscultating the fetal heart rate every fifteen minutes and encouraging Barb to change positions frequently.

When Barb began to feel the urge to push, the children were cleaned up and brought into the room. They all marvelled as the head, shoulders, and body of the baby appeared. The nurse-midwife eased out the baby's head and shoulders; Bob caught the baby and placed him on Barb's abdomen. The children tenderly touched their new brother. The nurse-midwife clamped and Bob cut the cord after it stopped pulsating. Barb's friend took pictures of the delighted children and the baby. The midwife left about two hours after the birth as her assessment of the mother and baby indicated both were in satisfactory condition. The RN stayed for four more hours and reported to the midwife before leaving. Bob planned to stay home for the next week to help take the baby to the pediatrician and to file a birth certificate at the city hall.

Review Question

Match the following with the appropriate birth setting:

1. _____ family provides some supplies
2. _____ stirrups
3. _____ modified labor room
4. _____ children at birth

a. traditional hospital setting
b. birthing room
c. alternative birth center
d. home

Answers

1. d. The family provides some supplies for a home birth.
2. a. Stirrups are commonly used in the traditional hospital setting.
3. b. A birthing room is often a modified labor room.
4. All but a. Children may be present at birth in a birth center or at home (and occasionally in a birthing room).

Advantages and Disadvantages of Each Birth Setting

THE TRADITIONAL HOSPITAL SETTING. In the last fifty years, the setting for childbirth has shifted from home to the hospital. In the traditional hospital setting, the woman labors in a labor room, delivers in a delivery room, and recovers in a recovery room.

Advantages of giving birth in the traditional hospital setting are:
1. Supervision is provided by skilled health care professionals.
2. Personnel and equipment are immediately available to handle complications or emergency situations.
3. Established procedures provide a sense of security.
4. The presence of the husband or one other support person is allowed.

Disadvantages of giving birth in the traditional hospital setting are:
1. In all labors, obstetric intervention, such as the routine use of enemas, intravenous fluids, electronic fetal monitoring, and episiotomies, is often the rule.
2. The woman has little control over how her labor is managed by the hospital staff.
3. Iatrogenic disorders (resulting from the activity of a physician) may occur; for example, infection from invasive procedures; that is, repeated vaginal exams, internal electronic monitoring, and so forth.
4. The woman may be confined to bed and periodically separated from her support person.
5. Individualized care and continuity of care from the hospital staff may be lacking owing to staffing patterns; that is, one nurse for every three to four patients, and different nurses for labor, delivery, and recovery.
6. Privacy may be impaired by semiprivate labor rooms and numerous medical and nursing students.
7. Anxiety may be increased if the private physician is absent during labor, or if he arrives at the last minute for delivery.
8. The labor process is interrupted by the transfer to the delivery room.
9. Delivery is made more difficult by the lithotomy position (flat on back with legs up in stirrups).
10. A support person other than the husband is often denied entry to the delivery room. At times, even the husband is denied attendance at the birth.
11. Separation of the mother, father, and baby is customary shortly after birth.

Routines vary with each hospital and can often be modified if the woman communicates her preferences to the hospital staff. Transitions are occurring in varying degrees, including less medical intervention in the physiologic aspects of the childbirth experience. Several ways in which both can be accomplished will be presented later in this chapter.

THE BIRTHING ROOM. A birthing room is a homelike room located within the labor and delivery area of a hospital. The woman labors, gives birth, and recovers, using the same bed and room. Hospitals have developed birthing rooms as a result of consumer demands for a birth experience more personalized than is customary in the traditional hospital setting.

Advantages of giving birth in a birthing room are:
1. The atmosphere in a birthing room is warm and relaxing.
2. Privacy and continuous presence of the primary support person is safeguarded.
3. If possible, the same staff nurse provides individualized care throughout the entire labor, birth, and recovery.
4. Obstetric intervention is usually minimal.
5. The parents usually have discussed their preferences for their birth experience with their primary caregiver (physician or certified nurse-midwife) prior to admission.
6. Parents have immediate and prolonged contact with their baby.
7. Trained personnel and emergency equipment are immediately available if a complication arises.
8. Home visits by nurses are sometimes provided following early discharge.

Disadvantages of giving birth in a birthing room are:
1. The presence of friends, relatives, or children (other than the primary support person) may be restricted during labor and birth owing to space limitations and hospital policy.
2. Often the woman is admitted to the birthing room only if she is in active labor, if her primary caregiver is present, or if staffing is adequate.
3. Since obstetric technology is readily available, precautionary intervention such as the use of IVs and monitors may occur even if it is not absolutely necessary.
4. The length of time spent with the baby after birth varies, and separation of the family may occur if the woman is transferred to a traditional recovery room.

Hospital rules and routines regarding use of a birthing room vary widely. Some hospitals allow only women who remain low risk (complication free) throughout their pregnancy to give birth in a birthing room; if complications arise during labor or birth, the woman is transferred to the traditional labor or delivery room for care. Other hospitals use birthing rooms for the majority of their women, using procedures such as induction and monitoring in the birthing room if necessary, and transferring the woman to a delivery room only for operative deliveries, which require anesthesia.

THE ALTERNATIVE BIRTH CENTER. An alternative birth center (ABC) is a maternity care facility located outside, but nearby, a hospital. The woman labors, gives birth, and recovers in a homelike setting. ABCs have been established in an attempt to decrease the rising incidence of home births. They provide a safe alternative to home delivery by combining the comforts of home with the safety features of a hospital.

Advantages of giving birth in a birth center are:
1. Individualized, family-centered care is given by an experienced professional staff.
2. Friends, relatives, and children are welcome if the woman desires.
3. A separate family room is available for early labor, or for visitors, if the parents desire privacy in the bedroom.
4. Parents have control over their birth experience with intervention from the staff only as needed.
5. There is no separation of the family after birth.
6. Early discharge facilitating family integration takes place within 24 hours.
7. Professional follow-up care is provided during the first few postpartum days.
8. Equipment, such as oxygen, Ambu bags, intravenous fluids, and Pitocin and other drugs, is available to meet immediate needs if a complication arises.
9. Emergency transportation is provided, as well as back-up care by a physician in a hospital.

Disadvantages of giving birth in an alternative birth center are:
1. Transfer to a hospital is necessary for on-going care if a complication arises. Time lost during transfer to a hospital may be life-threatening.*
2. Some women consider early discharge to be a disadvantage and choose to give birth in a hospital birthing room instead, so that they may rest in the hospital for a few days before returning home.

In-hospital alternative birth centers have also been established. They vary from a birthing room in that the family stays in the same room for the remainder of the hospital stay, which is usually 24 hours. Thus, the mother can get some rest, the family can remain together, and the time lost during transfer to the traditional labor and delivery area if a complication arises is minimized.

---

*No actual cases of critical emergency transfers or deaths during transfer from a birth center to a hospital have been reported in the literature.

THE HOME BIRTH. Home birth is one of the most controversial issues in childbirth today. Increasing numbers of couples are having their children at home.

Advantages of giving birth at home are:
1. The parents have maximum control over their birth experience; the risk of intervention is minimal.
2. An intimate atmosphere can prevail in the familiar setting, facilitating relaxation for all present.
3. Labor does not have to be interrupted by a trip to the hospital or birth center.
4. The parents decide who will be present at the birth, including friends, relatives, and children.
5. No separation of the family occurs after birth.

Disadvantages of giving birth at home are:
1. Because home births are not approved by the majority of the established medical community, a woman may have difficulty finding a qualified health care professional to give prenatal care and to attend the birth.
2. Medical supplies necessary to meet immediate emergency needs of the mother or baby may not be available.
3. Back-up emergency care by a physician in a hospital may be difficult to arrange in advance.
4. Transfer to a hospital can be life-threatening if the hospital is not located near the home, or if emergency care is not available during the transfer.

The birth attendant (the person who assists with the actual delivery) at a home birth varies from the father of the baby or a friend or a relative, to a lay-midwife, certified nurse-midwife, or physician. Whatever the status may be, the birth attendant must have the necessary knowledge, skills, and supplies to detect complications and to respond appropriately. A complication such as fetal distress can be life-threatening but need not be if the birth attendant correctly intervenes immediately.

The advantages and disadvantages of each birth setting listed on the previous pages are not all inclusive, nor are they limited to each particular setting. The atmosphere in the traditional hospital setting *can* be warm and relaxed, while the atmosphere at a home birth can become tense. Parents *can* have control over how the birth of their baby is managed and can control how much contact they will have with their baby after birth in the traditional hospital setting. Much depends on the attitude of the parents and the personnel in each setting, rather than on the setting itself.

Review Questions

Answer *true* or *false* to the following statements:

_____ 1. Prolonged contact with the baby immediately after birth is customary in the traditional hospital setting.

_____ 2. The parents decide who will be present at birth in the traditional hospital setting.

_____ 3. Women who labor in a birthing room give birth in a delivery room.

_____ 4. Personnel and equipment are available in an alternative birth center to meet most immediate emergency needs.

_____ 5. A woman may have difficulty finding a qualified health care professional to attend a home birth.

Answers

1. False.   Separation of the mother, father, and baby is customary shortly after birth in the traditional hospital setting.
2. False.   The presence of visitors other than the primary support person is usually not allowed during labor and delivery in the traditional hospital setting.
3. False.   The woman labors, delivers, and recovers in the same bed in a birthing room.
4. True.   Personnel and equipment are available in an alternative birth center to meet most immediate emergency needs.
5. True.   A woman may have difficulty finding a qualified health care professional to attend a home birth.

Candidates for Nontraditional Birth Settings

While most women can give birth safely in nontraditional settings, some will need the medical expertise and equipment available only in the traditional hospital setting. Therefore, all women planning to give birth in a nontraditional setting should be screened throughout their pregnancy and labor and should remain at low risk for the occurrence of complications.

History and laboratory results must be within normal limits. This means no evidence of the following:

hypertension	active syphilis or herpes
epilepsy	active tuberculosis

diabetes
heart disease
kidney disease
grand multiparity
previous cesarean delivery

Rh negative blood with positive
  antibody titers
severe anemia
severe psychiatric problems

In addition, the woman should be emotionally mature and stable and have the support of her significant other. Together they should prepare for the birth experience by reading and attending childbirth classes.

The pregnancy must be normal with no evidence of the following:
hydramnios
pre-eclampsia
multiple gestation
pre- or postmaturity
abnormal presentation or lie

abnormal vaginal bleeding
congenital anomalies
inappropriate weight gain or size for
  gestational age

Spontaneous labor should begin within 24 hours after rupture of membranes. The woman must agree to transfer of self and/or baby to the hospital (or out of birthing room), if complications occur during the labor, birth, or early postpartum period.

If any of the following complications occur during labor, transfer to the traditional hospital setting should occur:
thick meconuim staining
fetal distress
prolapsed cord

prolonged labor
pre-eclampsia/eclampsia
abnormal vaginal bleeding

Transfer to a hospital may be necessary after the birth for:
retained placenta or placental
  fragments
third or fourth degree lacerations

hemorrhage
newborn complications

The presence of any *one* factor may not automatically exclude the mother from giving birth in a nontraditional setting, but it does necessitate careful and continuous assessment.

Review Questions

1. Which of the following conditions are contraindications to giving birth in a nontraditional setting?
    a. Rh positive blood in the mother
    b. maternal heart disease
    c. vertex presentation
    d. previous cesarean delivery
    e. lack of support from significant other

2. Which of the following complications occurring during labor, delivery, or the early postpartum period necessitate transfer to the traditional hospital setting?
   a. bloody show
   b. fetal distress
   c. retained placenta
   d. first degree laceration
   e. prolapsed cord

Answers

1. b, d, e. Maternal heart disease, previous cesarean delivery, and lack of support from significant other are contraindications to giving birth in a nontraditional setting.
2. b, c, e. Fetal distress, retained placenta, and prolapsed cord necessitate transfer to the traditional hospital setting.

The Role of the Nurse

Since birth settings vary widely from one geographic area to another, nurses should be aware of what alternatives are available in their community. They should examine their personal feelings about various birth settings and be able to provide unbiased, factual information about the advantages and disadvantages of each setting.

The nurse should encourage expectant couples to explore the alternatives available to them. This can be done through reading, attending classes, touring hospitals and alternative birth centers, and communicating with health care professionals and couples who have used any of the various birth settings. The decision of where to have a baby is a very personal one, but the nurse can assist the couple to make a responsible, informed decision.

Ideally, all parents should have a variety of nontraditional birthing options, each offering safe, quality care. Nurses can become involved with other qualified health care professionals and consumers in providing these alternatives.

ALTERNATIVE PRACTICES DURING LABOR AND BIRTH

The alternatives described here will help the reader to facilitate the natural, physiologic process of childbirth, as well as to meet the psychologic needs of the woman. These alternatives to traditional labor and delivery practices are adaptable to the woman in labor in any birth setting; in some areas of the United States they are already routinely implemented.

The First Stage of Labor

EARLY LABOR ROUTINES. Admission to the hospital can be an anxiety provoking experience for the woman in labor, particularly if she is separated from her support person. Couples can avoid separation on admission to the hospital by preregistering during the last trimester of pregnancy. Upon admission to the labor room, the nurse should give the support person the choice of remaining in the room or waiting in a lounge. The very presence of the partner can help the woman feel more comfortable and relaxed in the new, unfamiliar setting. As the admission procedures are being done, the nurse can elicit the couple's preferences or plans for the experience of childbirth.

Shaving the perineal hair was once thought to prevent infection, but extensive studies[1] have disproved this. Alternatives to the traditional perineal shave include leaving the hair as is, clipping the hair if it is long, or clipping the hair only in the perineal region. Clipping may be done at home by the mother. The perineal area should be cleansed of vaginal secretions (amniotic fluid, bloody show) as needed during labor and immediately prior to the birth.

An enema is often unnecessary as frequent loose stools may occur at the onset of labor. If the woman has not had a bowel movement in the past 24 hours, or if stool is felt in the rectum, a small enema (e.g., Fleet) is sufficient to cleanse the lower bowel of stool. The enema may be self-administered at home. (See Chapter 5 for contraindications to enemas.)

Early labor should be spent in restful activity. The woman may walk around, visit with family or friends, watch TV, play cards or other games, or lounge on a couch or rocking chair. The nurse should suggest or encourage these activities, unless the mother is tired and needs to sleep. If the membranes are ruptured and the presenting part is unengaged, her activity may be confined to bed to prevent prolapse of the cord. The woman should be allowed to eat lightly and drink fluids to replenish her energy. Any clothing that is clean and comfortable may be worn. Many women prefer their street clothes, gown, or robe as a means of maintaining their personal identity.

Review Questions

1. What action can the couple take to avoid separation on admission to the hospital? _____

    _____

    _____

2. What action can the nurse take to minimize anxiety on admission to the labor room? _____

_____

_____

3. List two alternatives to the traditional perineal shave.
   a. _____
   b. _____

4. Identify two situations when a small enema may be needed.
   a. _____
   b. _____

5. Name three activities the nurse can encourage the woman to do in early labor.
   a. _____
   b. _____
   c. _____

6. Identify two situations in early labor that warrant confinement to bed.
   a. _____
   b. _____

Answers

1. To avoid separation on admission to the hospital, the couple can preregister during the last trimester of pregnancy.

2. To minimize anxiety on admission to the labor room, the nurse can give the support person the choice of remaining in the room or waiting in a lounge.

3. Alternatives to the traditional perineal shave are (a) not shaving, (b) clipping long hair, and (c) clipping the hair only in the perineal region.

4. A small enema may be needed if (a) the woman has not had a bowel movement in the past 24 hours, and (b) if stool is felt in the rectum.

5. The nurse can encourage women in early labor to (a) walk around, (b) watch TV, (c) eat lightly and drink as desired, (d) visit with family or friends, (e) play cards or other games, and (f) lounge on a couch or rocking chair.

6. The nurse should not encourage activity other than at bedside when: (a) the woman is tired and needs to sleep, and (b) the membranes are ruptured and the presenting part is unengaged, since a prolapsed cord could result.

FAMILY AND FRIENDS. Many women feel more comfortable and relaxed during labor if they are attended by familiar people. Some women choose to have present a *monitrice* (a labor coach trained in the Lamaze method), a close female friend, their mother, children, or other family members or friends, in addition to their partner. Everyone present *should* be there to *support* the woman's efforts to give birth. If some of the people present are spectators, just watching and waiting for the baby to be born, the woman may feel pressured to perform.

In those hospital settings in which only one support person is permitted, the support of the same nurse throughout the entire birth process is desirable. Too often the woman and her partner are assisted in labor by a number of nurses giving conflicting advice; then the woman is cared for by a different delivery room nurse who is busy assisting the doctor and completing the delivery room record; and then she is cared for by a different recovery room nurse who has little idea of what the mother has just experienced. It is difficult for a nurse to give a woman personalized care in the delivery or recovery room unless she has been with her throughout the labor experience.

The presence of children at the birth may or may not be desirable. Many people say children may be too young to understand and can easily misinterpret their mother's expressions of stress and pain. Some feel that young children are not disciplined enough to keep from interfering and placing demands on their mother even during labor. Others recommend that siblings not be present at birth because the long-term effects are uncertain.[2] Advocates of children at birth feel that children who are actively involved in the pregnancy, labor, and birth welcome the new sibling more openly and show less sibling rivalry and regression than those who are not. Childbirth is considered a normal part of the life experience to be shared by the entire family.

Children who are present at birth should be well prepared for what to expect—the hard work, the sounds, the pain, the blood, the nudity, and the appearance of the baby and the placenta. They should be familiar with the birthplace. They should know what they can do (get Mommy ice, juice, wet washcloths, and so forth), and what they cannot do (interrupt Mommy during a contraction, ask Daddy to read, and so forth). Children need their own support person at this time, someone who has no other responsibilities than to be sensitive to the children's needs and to meet them. Children must also have the freedom to leave the birth setting; a separate family room or a yard in which to play is usually available at home or in a birth center. Since the environment of an unfamiliar or small birthing room may be threatening to a child, an alternative is for someone to bring the child to the hospital immediately after the birth so that the family can still be together in the first few hours after birth. In this situation, parents may find that boys are initially more interested in exploring the room, while girls may be immediately attentive to mother and baby.

When expectant parents prepare for the presence of friends and family at the birth of their baby, they should also prepare for the birth without them present. Sometimes women change their minds during labor and prefer to have only their partner present. If the children become disruptive or choose to leave on their own out of fear or boredom, the parents should be accepting. Sometimes, just for logistical reasons (the late night, distance, and so forth) it is not possible to get the others to the birth. Sometimes complications arise, such as those described in the earlier part of this chapter, that necessitate transfer to the hospital and subsequent exclusion of others from the birth.

Review Questions

1. Everyone present at a birth should be there to _____
    _____
    _____

2. In hospital settings in which only one support person is permitted, a desirable alternative is: _____
    _____
    _____

3. Give two arguments *against* children at birth.
    a. _____
    b. _____

4. Give two arguments *for* children at birth.
    a. _____
    b. _____

5. Children who are present at birth should:
    a. _____
    b. _____
    c. _____

Answers

1. Everyone present at a birth should be there to support the woman, not just watch and wait for the baby to be born.

2. In hospital settings in which only one support person is permitted, the support of the same nurse throughout the entire birth process is desirable.

3. Arguments *against* children at birth are:
    a. they can easily misinterpret the mother's expressions of stress and pain.
    b. they are not disciplined enough to keep from interfering and placing demands on their mother.
    c. long-term effects are uncertain.
4. Arguments *for* children at birth are:
    a. they welcome the new sibling more openly.
    b. they show less sibling rivalry and regression.
    c. birth is a normal life experience to be shared by family members.
5. Children at birth should:
    a. be prepared for what to expect.
    b. be familiar with the birthplace.
    c. know their privileges and restrictions.
    d. have their own support person.
    e. have the freedom to leave the setting.

POSITIONS DURING ACTIVE LABOR. As contractions become more uncomfortable, the woman in labor usually puts aside her cards or shuts off the TV and lies down in bed. Many women lie down in bed merely because they think that is what is expected of them. Lying flat on the back can lead to maternal supine hypotension, fetal bradycardia and acidosis, less effective uterine contractions, longer labor, and greater discomfort for the mother. Therefore, if the woman chooses to be in bed, she should sit up or lie on her side with her head elevated at least 30 degrees. Although it is unlikely that a woman would choose to remain in the same position throughout labor, she should be encouraged to change position approximately every half hour. Position *changes* may be more important than a single best position.[3]

The woman need not be confined to bed. She may benefit from ambulating, standing, kneeling, or sitting. Experimental studies cited by Noble[4] on positions during labor show that ambulation shortens the duration of labor, decreases the need for analgesics and oxytocin, and decreases the incidence of fetal heart rate abnormalities. The standing position also has the potential for greater intimacy and interaction between the woman and her partner, as there are no physical barriers (e.g., bed, chair) between them. The woman can lean against her partner for support during contractions, and the partner or nurse can massage her arms, back, sacrum, or any other part of the body that needs relaxing (Fig. 9-1).

Another beneficial position during labor is kneeling with her arms and upper portion of the body leaning forward, resting on a bed or chair (Fig. 9-2). A pillow or folded blanket should be placed on the floor under the knees for added comfort. This position is particularly effective if the fetus is OP or OT, because it relieves pressure on the sacrum and may

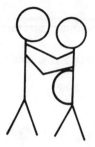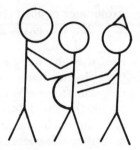

Figure 9-1. (*Left*) Partner and woman; (*Right*) partner, woman, and nurse.

help to rotate the fetus. The woman can easily do pelvic rocking in this position, and the partner or nurse can massage her back and shoulders using lotion or powder, or apply counterpressure or warm compresses to her sacrum. Many women find this kneeling position less inhibiting and easier for breathing than getting on all fours.

Sitting can also be comfortable for the woman in labor. The woman can sit on a chair, a bean bag, a stuffed recliner, or on the side of the bed with legs dangling, or in bed with pillows to support her back. The partner can sit at the head of the bed with the woman sitting between his legs, leaning back against him for support (Fig. 9-3). In experimental studies cited by Roberts,[5] contractions were found to be more effective when sitting than when supine; however, contractions were of lower intensity and less effective in cervical dilation than when in the standing or lateral position.

Review Questions

Answer *true* or *false* to the following statements.

1. _____ Lying flat on the back can cause maternal supine hypotension and fetal bradycardia.

2. _____ If a woman is comfortable, she may remain in one position throughout labor.

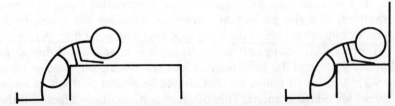

Figure 9-2. (*Left*) Woman and bed; (*Right*) woman and chair.

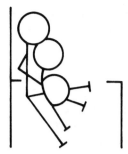

Figure 9-3. Partner and woman sitting in bed.

3. _____ Ambulation lengthens labor and increases the need for analgesics.

4. _____ Lying flat on the back helps rotate a fetus from an OP or OT position.

5. _____ Contractions are most effective in the sitting position.

Answers

1. True.   Lying flat can cause maternal supine hypotension and fetal bracycardia.

2. False. A woman in labor should change positions approximately every half hour.

3. False. Ambulation shortens labor and decreases the need for analgesics.

4. False. Lying flat on the back does not help rotate a fetus from the OP or OT position.

5. False. Contractions are more effective in the standing or lateral position than in a sitting position.

BREATHING AND RELAXING. A very popular method of dealing with the increasingly uncomfortable contractions of labor is the psychoprophylactic or Lamaze method of childbirth. Women prepared in this method respond to each contraction by concentrating intently on breathing according to a set pattern and on consciously relaxing the muscles not involved in labor. (See Chapter 8.) This conditioned response helps the woman block out the painful sensations of labor.

Some critics of the Lamaze approach are opposed to the techniques of distraction, disassociation, and control. They feel that these techniques can be physiologically threatening by causing undue physical exertion and fatigue, and psychologically threatening by setting the woman up for failure if she cannot perform according to the set pattern. Advocates of a "let go and flow" approach believe that a woman should listen to and interpret messages from her body rather than control or disregard them. They emphasize relaxation throughout labor, letting the breath flow at its natural rhythm, and doing what feels right for the individual. This approach also requires preparation as the woman must gain knowledge of the process of labor and develop a trust in her body during pregnancy in order to let go at the time of birth.

Just as there is no single best position for labor, there is no one best response to the contractions of labor. The nurse should determine what specific preparation a woman has for labor and what her expectations are of herself and others. With such knowledge and an open attitude, the nurse can support the couple in the way they desire, helping to adapt the techniques learned in class to the situation at hand.

Music may facilitate relaxation during active labor, particularly if it is music the woman has chosen and has practiced breathing and relaxing to during her pregnancy. Most birth centers and birthing rooms have a radio or stereo available, but the couple may have to bring their own radio or cassette player to the traditional hospital labor room. They are usually responsible for any personal items they bring in.

Another alternative related to relaxation during active labor is the use of a warm shower or a clean bath tub filled deep with water. These can be an effective substitute for pain medication. They can also be used to break the monotony of a long labor. A shower may be given instead of a bath if the membranes are ruptured. Lower back pain may be relieved by directing the water to flow over the lower back. Odent[6] feels that water helps the woman in labor reach a high level of relaxation and reduces her inhibitions, thereby allowing her to cooperate with the forces of labor. Brown[7] recommends that the bath be comfortably warm and cover the body completely. The bath may continue for as long as it is effective in assisting the woman to cope with the contractions. The woman in labor should never be left alone while in the tub and should be assisted out of the tub periodically to monitor the fetal heart rate and cervical dilatation and for the birth of the baby.

Review Question

1. List two alternatives to facilitate relaxation during active labor.
    a. _____
    b. _____

Answer

1. Alternatives to facilitate relaxation during active labor are:
    a. "let go and flow" approach
    b. music that the woman has chosen or practiced with.
    c. warm water during a bath or shower.

FLUIDS—ORAL AND INTRAVENOUS. Fluids and nutrients are essential during active labor as the woman is working and expanding energy; without them she will become thirsty, and possibly hypoglycemic and dehydrated. Most women prefer something to drink, rather than eat, during active labor. Liquids such as water, soft drinks, fruit juices, bouillon, or teas may be taken as desired. Hard candy, suckers, ice chips, popsicles, and glycerine swabs may also be used to relieve a dry, unpleasant taste in the mouth. If the woman takes little fluid orally, vomits repeatedly, or if labor is prolonged, fluids may need to be given intravenously. If the labor is complicated and a cesarean birth is anticipated, oral fluids are usually withheld.

Review Questions

1. What besides liquids may be given to relieve a dry, unpleasant taste?
    a. _____
    b. _____
    c. _____

2. When may intravenous fluids be needed?
    a. _____
    b. _____
    c. _____

Answers

1. Besides liquids, the following may be given to relieve a dry, unpleasant taste: (a) hard candy or suckers; (b) ice chips, (c) popsicles, and (d) glycerine swabs.

2. Intravenous fluids may be needed when:
    (a) the woman takes little fluids orally,
    (b) the woman vomits repeatedly,
    (c) labor is prolonged,
    (d) labor is complicated and a cesarean birth is anticipated.

FETAL HEART RATE MONITORING. Experts agree that the single most informative parameter of fetal well-being during labor is the fetal heart rate (see Chapter 2); but there is controversy regarding the best method of monitoring. Advocates of electronic fetal monitoring (EFM) say that its use reduces the incidence of stillbirths, mental retardation, and cerebral palsy. They feel that labor poses a potential threat to every fetus and that constant electronic monitoring of the fetal heart rate is necessary to recognize fetal distress. To the contrary, studies cited by Ettner[8] show no difference in infant outcome whether electronically monitored or auscultated with a fetoscope; internal EFM does result in more postpartum endometritis and occasional newborn scalp abscesses. Critics also oppose limitations of mobility, early and artificial rupture of membranes (to apply an internal lead), potential maternal anxiety, and increased cesarean delivery rate associated with EFM.[9]

Because the benefits of EFM do not clearly outweigh the risks, many feel that routine EFM should be limited to high-risk women. In 1979, a National Institute of Health Task Force on Predictors of Fetal Distress found periodic auscultation of the FHR to be an acceptable method of assessment of fetal condition for low-risk women. They defined periodic auscultation to include auscultation of the FHR every 15 minutes during the first stage of labor and every 5 minutes during the second stage; in both cases, a period of 30 seconds following a contraction is required. Use of a Doppler is preferred, because unlike a fetoscope, it effectively transmits the FHR through the contracting uterus, regardless of the maternal position. It also informs and reassures parents of the fetal condition, facilitating their cooperation when intervention proves necessary.

An alternative method of fetal monitoring uses radiotelemetry to transmit the fetal heart and intrauterine pressure. A device placed intravaginally transmits signals to a receiving and data read-out apparatus. The main advantage of radiotelemetric fetal monitoring is that it allows the woman to move freely and ambulate at variable distances from the radio receiver.

Review Questions

Answer *true* or *false* to the following statements:

1. _____ Research studies clearly demonstrate improved fetal outcome with EFM.

2. _____ Risks associated with EFM include increased cesarean delivery rates and more postpartum endometritis.

Answers

1. False.   Studies are not conclusive about improved fetal outcome with EFM.

2. True.   EFM increases cesarean delivery rates and postpartum endometritis.

The Second Stage of Labor

POSITIONS FOR PUSHING. The nurse can facilitate descent of the fetus during the second stage of labor through proper positioning and pushing techniques. The common practice of instructing the woman to lie flat on her back, placing her hands under her thighs, and pulling back as she pushes (a) requires the woman to push against gravity, (b) increases the tension of the lower extremities and pelvic floor, (c) diminishes the physical dimensions of the pelvis, and (d) uses the abdominal muscles to lift the upper torso, detracting from their primary function of pushing the baby out.

Alternative positions the nurse can help the woman assume are:

1.   The "C" position: sitting propped up with the spine curved like a rainbow, the knees bent, the legs relaxed and apart, and the feet flat on the bed. The woman may be propped up by using pillows or a back-rest, by elevating the head of the bed at least 45 degrees, or by leaning against her partner who is sitting at the head of the bed;
2.   side-lying with upper leg bent and raised;
3.   up on hands and knees;
4.   sitting on the toilet with a sheet under the seat and over the bowl to insure safety;
5.   squatting, which enlarges the pelvic outlet and allows for more efficient bearing down efforts. Squatting requires a great deal of energy and will probably necessitate someone supporting the woman under her shoulders, or the woman holding onto a chair or siderail. (Fig. 9-4). The woman may also need help to assume a comfortable resting position between contractions, such as leaning against her partner, or sitting on the chair or bed. Sitting on a birthing stool simulates the squatting position and requires less energy. The woman can remain on the stool between contractions, leaning against pillows or her partner for support, and stretching out her legs between contractions to avoid cramping.

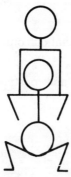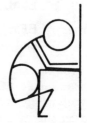

Figure 9-4. (*Left*) Squatting with shoulder support; (*Right*) squatting with chair support.

Review Questions

1. Two disadvantages of pushing while lying flat on the back with legs pulled towards the body are:
   a. _____
   b. _____

2. Three alternative positions for pushing are:
   a. _____
   b. _____
   c. _____

3. Two ways to support a woman in the squatting position are:
   a. _____
   b. _____

Answers

1. Pushing while lying flat with legs pulled towards the body:
   a. requires the woman to push against gravity,
   b. increases tension on the lower extremities and pelvic floor,
   c. diminishes the physical dimensions of the pelvis, and
   d. uses the abdominal muscles to lift the upper torso, detracting from their primary function of pushing the baby out.

2. Alternative positions for pushing are: (a) the "C" position, (b) side-lying, (c) up on hands and knees, (d) sitting on shielded toilet, and (e) squatting.

3. Ways to support a woman in the squatting position are:
   (a) holding her under the shoulders,
   (b) having her hold onto a chair or siderail,
   (c) sitting on a birthing stool.

PUSHING TECHNIQUES. The traditional method of pushing with prolonged breath-holding and bearing down with maximum force can be detrimental to mother and fetus. Reduced cardiac output that results from sustained breath-holding, along with maternal acidosis resulting from exertion, may contribute to fetal hypoxia.

An alternative to the traditional method of pushing is *exhale breathing* (also called *forced exhalation*). Using this method, the nurse instructs the woman to bear down only when the expulsive urge is irresistible. The woman inhales, holds her breath, contracts her abdominal muscles, and pushes while exhaling slowly and lightly through slightly pursed lips. During the next inhalation of air, which usually occurs in six to seven seconds, she concentrates on keeping the abdominal muscles contracted, thereby maintaining the progress made in fetal descent. (More details are given in the McKay article in the American Journal of Nursing, 1981.) Because the second stage of labor may be lengthened with the use of exhale breathing, particularly for the primigravida, this technique has been greeted with less than enthusiastic support by many health care providers. Yet, in a study by Cohen,[10] no significant increase in the frequency of perinatal mortality, neonatal morbidity, or low five-minute Apgar scores was noted with long second stages.

A single method for pushing is unlikely to work for every woman during the second stage of labor. The amount of maternal effort and time required will depend on the particular circumstances of the labor, for example, size and position of the fetus or parity of the woman. The nurse can encourage spontaneous individualized *pushing* styles by giving the mother the following *guidelines:*

a. Assume a comfortable, gravity-assisted position (as described in the previous section).
b. Push in the direction of the vagina, not the rectum.
c. Contract only the abdominal muscles; keep the rest of the body, especially the face, thighs, and pelvic floor, relaxed.
d. Inhale, hold the breath, and push as long and as hard as the urge is felt, letting out air or sound if desired.
e. Keep the abdominal muscles contracted when inhaling between pushes.
f. Pant to control the urge to push at the time of birth.

Some women will push more effectively if they can view or touch their baby as it emerges from the birth canal. By using a mirror or encouraging the mother to touch her baby's head as it crowns (appears at the vaginal orifice), the mother can see or feel the effectiveness of her efforts. Some women are inhibited in their pushing efforts because of extreme rectal pressure. The nurse can counteract this feeling by applying firm pressure against the rectum toward the vagina, using warm moist compresses. The fear of or actual defecation can also be inhibiting; the nurse can reassure the woman that this is a normal occurrence.

Review Questions

Choose the correct response(s).
1. The nurse can facilitate spontaneous, individual pushing styles by encouraging the mother to:
    a. assume a comfortable, gravity-assisted position,
    b. push even though she does not feel the urge,
    c. hold her breath for at least 15 seconds and give three good pushes with each contraction,
    d. pant, not push, at the time of birth.

2. The nurse can facilitate effective pushing by:
    a. positioning a mirror for the mother to see,
    b. encouraging the mother to touch her baby's head as it crowns,
    c. applying firm pressure against the symphysis pubis to counter-act the rectal pressure,
    d. applying cold compresses to the rectal area.

Answers

1. a, d. The nurse can encourage the mother to assume a comfortable gravity-assisted position; push as long and as hard as she feels the urge to; and pant at the time of birth.

2. a, b. Effective pushing can be facilitated by seeing and feeling the positive results and by providing counterpressure on the rectal region using warm compresses.

GIVING BIRTH—LABOR ROOM vs. DELIVERY ROOM. Giving birth in the labor room rather than moving to a delivery room has the advantage of not interfering with or disrupting the progress of labor. The woman is free to continue pushing and assume any position she desires for the birth of her baby. She does not have to readjust to a new and often anxiety producing environment and possibly new personnel who may not be acquainted with her and her labor. Portable equipment for the birth and emergencies can be available in the labor room.

If transfer to the delivery room is to take place, the nurse can mini-mize the couple's stress by keeping them together and by making the transfer early enough so that the woman does not have to resist the urge to push during the procedure. Side-lying during transfer prevents mater-nal supine hypotension and diminishes the urge to push. Once on the delivery table, the nurse should prop the woman up in a semisitting posi-tion using pillows or a pie-shaped wedge. This position facilitates pushing with the force of gravity and enables the woman to participate more actively in the birth. Stirrups, if used, should be low to prevent unnecessary tension on the perineum. Alternative delivery approaches are to (a) break the delivery table only halfway so that the woman can rest her feet far apart on the lower end of the table, (b) move the labor bed into the delivery room, and (c) deliver in a side-lying position with the upper leg elevated. A few delivery rooms are equipped with an adjustable birthing chair instead of a delivery table.

Review Questions

1. Two nursing actions that minimize a couple's stress during transfer to the delivery room are:
   a. _____
   b. _____

2. How should the woman and the stirrups be positioned on the delivery table? _____
   _____

3. Describe two alternative delivery approaches.
   a. _____
   b. _____

Answers

1. Nursing actions that minimize the couple's stress during transfer to the delivery room are:
   a. keeping the couple together
   b. timing the transfer so that the woman does not have to resist the urge to push.
   c. having the woman assume side-lying position to decrease the urge to push.

2. The woman should be in semisitting position on the delivery table; stirrups, if used, should be low.

3. Alternative delivery approaches are to (a) break the delivery table only halfway, (b) move the labor bed into the delivery room, and (c) deliver in a side-lying position.

THE INTACT PERINEUM. The need for an episiotomy can be minimized by avoiding the lithotomy position, by having the birth attendant support the perineum, and by having the woman control the urge to push. If the baby's head is slowly eased out at the end of or in between contractions, no episiotomy may be necessary and no lacerations may occur. The nurse can help the woman maintain control as the baby's head is born by speaking softly, yet distinctly near her ear with specific directions. She should prepare the woman for a burning sensation as the perineal tissue stretches around the baby's head. Massaging the perineum with oil (wheat germ or Vitamin E oil) or using warm compresses as crowning takes place helps the perineum to relax. Daily perineal massage during late pregnancy increases circulation to the perineal muscles. This optimizes tissue integrity and elasticity, contributing to the ability to stretch without tearing. A technique for perineal massage is described by Schrag in the Journal of Nurse-Midwifery.[11]

Review Question

1. List three actions that minimize the need for an episiotomy.
   a. _____
   b. _____
   c. _____

Answer

1. Actions that minimize the need for an episiotomy are:
   a. avoiding the lithotomy position,
   b. supporting the perineum,
   c. controlling the urge to push,
   d. slowly easing the baby's head out at the end of or in between contractions,
   e. preparing the mother for a burning sensation,
   f. massaging the perineum with oil during crowning,
   g. using warm compresses during crowning,
   h. massaging the perineum daily during late pregnancy.

GENTLE BIRTH. Frederick Leboyer, a French obstetrician, advocates gentle birth in his book entitled *Birth Without Violence*. According to Leboyer, attempts can be made after delivery to simulate the intrauterine environment, thereby minimizing the trauma of being born. Leboyer's method is to ease, not tug, the baby out into a quiet, dimly lit room. He is placed belly down on his mother's abdomen and is allowed to breathe on his own without painful stimuli. He is given a back massage as the cord stops pulsating, at which time the cord is cut. He is placed in a warm tub of water (usually by the father) to reassure the baby that his extrauterine environment is not a drastic change. He is then dried and returned to his mother for cuddling, stroking, and nursing.

Although specific techniques advocated by Leboyer such as low lights and delayed cord cutting have been criticized, his concept of treating the newborn as a uniquely sensitive human being has made considerable impact on birth practices.

Review Question

1. What is Leboyer's main concept? _____
_____
_____

Answer

1. Leboyer's main concept is to treat the newborn as an uniquely sensitive human being.

PROMOTING ATTACHMENT. The time immediately following birth is thought to be a sensitive period in the development of parent-infant attachment. An attachment, or bond, is "a unique relationship between two people that is specific and endures through time."[12] Even though a certain attachment to the fetus develops during pregnancy, the emergence of the infant at birth adds an entirely new dimension to the parent-infant relationship. Now there is an individual that the parents must get acquainted with, explore, identify, and claim as their own. Providing time for parents to interact with their infant in the first hours and days after birth will help parents begin this essential process.

To promote parent-infant interaction at the time of birth, the birth attendant can place the baby directly on the mother's bare abdomen. In some cases, the mother may wish to reach down, after the baby's head and shoulders are born, and lift the baby up on to her abdomen. In other cases, the father may wish to catch the baby. The baby should be placed on his stomach with the head lower than the chest to facilitate drainage of secretions from the nose and mouth. Gentle suctioning and tactile stimulation to initiate respirations, if necessary, can be done while on the mother's abdomen. The nurse should dry the baby to prevent heat loss via evaporation, and place a warm dry blanket over the mother and baby. A radiant heat warmer, if available, can also be placed over them. The father, or mother, may cut the cord.

If the newborn is given to the nurse by the birth attendant, she should present the baby to the parents as soon as he is dry and breathing well. Further physical care, such as identification procedures, can be postponed until the parents seem ready for an interruption (but must be completed before the mother and baby leave the delivery area).

The nurse should encourage the mother (and father) to become acquainted with her baby by touching, talking, and looking at him. She explores his body with her fingertips, first on the infant's extremities, followed by palm contact of the trunk, and finally enfolding him in her arms, holding him close to her body. She speaks to her baby in a high-pitched voice which the newborn prefers to a male voice. Immediately after birth and for about one hour afterwards, the baby is in a quiet, alert state; his eyes are open and he looks around, showing a preference for the human face. To promote eye-to-eye contact, the nurse should encourage the mother to sit up (conditions permitting) and hold the infant in the crook of her arm, eight to nine inches from her face. The nurse can postpone the instillation of an eye prophylaxis, which blurs the infant's vision, until after the parents have established eye-to-eye contact with their baby. (Most states require by law that newborn eye prophylaxis be given within one to two hours after birth to prevent ophthalmia neonatorum).

The nurse can also assist the mother to breastfeed when the baby shows rooting activity. Breastfeeding provides colostrum for the baby and stimulates oxytocin production in the mother. This promotes uterine contractions and may eliminate the need for IV oxytocin after the delivery of the placenta. The newborn will commonly lick the areola as though tasting prior to nursing. The nurse should reassure the mother that this is typical and in a few minutes her baby will nurse. Knowing this will prevent a feeling of uncertainity on the part of the mother regarding her ability to nurse her infant.

The opportunity for extended early contact with the infant may be particularly important for the father who, unlike the mother, may not be biologically or culturally primed to be responsive to infant cues.[13] Early contact of the father with the infant is significant in his becoming engrossed in the infant (a feeling of preoccupation, absorption, interest, and desire to touch, hold, and interact with the infant).[14] The nurse can place the baby in the father's arms when the mother seems ready to let go of the baby. Often new fathers will extend their arms to receive the baby in the palms of their hands, but the nurse can place the baby in the crook of his arm instead and encourage the father to hold the baby close.

The nurse must be sensitive to the parents' desire for interaction with their infant after birth. For parents who desire immediate and sustained contact with their baby, the nurse can provide this immediately after the birth and can offer the family the opportunity to remain together during the early postpartum period. For the mother who is too exhausted or uncomfortable to hold her newborn, the nurse can briefly unwrap the baby so the mother can inspect him visually and can encourage the father to hold the baby close to the mother so she can touch and kiss him. Each parent will proceed at his or her own pace in developing a relationship with the infant. The nurse should provide an opportunity for parent-infant interaction to occur but should not force it.

Review Question

1. Identify at least five actions the nurse can take to promote parent-infant attachment after birth.

   a. _____

   b. _____

   c. _____

   d. _____

   e. _____

Answer

1. The nurse can:
   a. present the baby to his parents as soon as he is dry and breathing well.
   b. encourage the mother to touch, talk to the baby, and establish eye-to-eye contact.
   c. postpone the instillation of eye prophylaxis, within the limits of the law.
   d. assist the mother to breastfeed.
   e. encourage the father to hold the baby.
   f. offer the family the opportunity to remain together during the early postpartum period.
   g. for tired mothers, unwrap the baby briefly; hold the baby close to the mother.

PICTURES AND CELEBRATIONS. Some women desire pictures or tape recordings of their birth experience. So much of the activity surrounding the birth is missed by the woman due to her intense concentration, both physically and mentally, on birthing the baby. Viewing pictures after the birth helps the woman to integrate this critical life experience into her total being. One woman expressed that she fell in love with her husband all over again when she fully realized, through viewing the pictures afterwards, how much he did for her during labor. In later years, the pictures can be used to explain pregnancy and birth to the child and can be especially helpful in preparing the child for the birth of a sibling.

If pictures are desired, it is recommended that they be taken by a person other than the primary support person and by one who is familiar with the birth process and the birth setting. The mother should let the photographer know, before labor's onset, what aspects of the birth to emphasize (e.g., mother's efforts, partner's role, or children's reactions) and what to leave out. Arrangements should also be made with caregivers in the particular birth setting beforehand.

Finally, birth is a joyous event that should be celebrated. Parents may wish to celebrate with food, wine, or champagne, a birthday party, prayer, or any other personal ceremony.

The Role of the Nurse—Summary

Prenatally, the nurse can help the expectant couple prepare for their baby's birth. The nurse should provide unbiased information on the alternatives available during the birth process and encourage clients to gain further information by reading and conversing with experienced couples and health care providers. By discussing advantages and disadvantages of various alternatives, the nurse can assist couples to decide which alternatives are desirable for them. The need to make mutually agreed upon arrangements with their primary caregiver *prior* to the onset of labor must be emphasized. Some childbirth educators recommend that the couple, in consultation with their primary caregiver, develop a written Birth Plan[15] to facilitate communication of their preferences with others at the place of birth. While preparing for a normal birth, the nurse should also provide information on alternatives if the labor deviates from the expected course.

During labor, the nurse should elicit the couple's preferences for the birth experience and genuinely attempt to provide them. If the couple does not communicate any preferences, the nurse should offer alternatives that will facilitate a safe, satisfying birth experience for them. Not all women desire or need the same type of care during labor and birth; thus the nurse must be aware of and respond to the individual needs of each expectant family.

Nurses must examine not only their own attitudes toward the management of birth, but also the written policies and routines of their health care facility. Nursing practice must be congruent with current knowledge and research findings. Nurses need to recognize that there are some deficiencies in the provision of care to expectant families and that nurses can be influential in modifying the present practices. By being attentive to the family's individual needs and desires during the birth process, nurses can promote a satisfying, self-fulfilling experience for each family member.

REFERENCES

1. PETTY, R: *Home Birth.* Domus Books, Chicago, 1979, p 51.

2. KLAUS, MH AND KENNELL, JH: *Parent-Infant Bonding,* ed 2. CV Mosby, St. Louis, 1982, p 127.

3. ROBERTS, J: *Alternative positions for childbirth. Part I: The first stage of labor.* J Nurse-Midwifery 25(4):11, 1980.

4. NOBLE, E: *Controversies in maternal effort during labor and delivery.* J Nurse-Midwifery 26(2):13, 1981.

5. ROBERTS, J: *Alternative positions for childbirth. Part I: The first stage of labor.* J Nurse-Midwifery 25(4):11, 1980.

6. ODENT, M: *The evolution of obstetrics at Pithiviers.* Birth Family J 8(1):7, 1981.

7. BROWN, C: *Therapeutic effects of bathing during labor.* J Nurse-Midwifery, 27(1):13, 1982.

8. ETTNER, FM: *Hospital obstetrics: Do the benefits outweigh the risks?* In STEWART, D AND STEWART, L (EDS): *21st Century Obstetrics Now!* Vol 1. NAPSAC, Inc, Marble Hill, Mo., 1978, p 148.

9. ETTNER, FM: *Hospital obstetrics: Do the benefits outweight the risks?* In STEWART, D AND STEWART, L (EDS): *21st Century Obstetrics Now!* Vol 1. NAPSAC, Inc, Marble Hill, Mo, 1978, pp 148–152.

10. COHEN, WR: *Influence of the duration of second stage labor on perinatal outcome and puerperal morbidity.* Obstet Gynecol, 49(3):266, 1977.

11. SCHRAG, K: *Maintenance of pelvic floor integrity during childbirth.* J Nurse-Midwifery, 24(6):26, 1979.

12. KLAUS, MH AND KENNELL, JH: *Parent-Infant Bonding,* ed 2. CV Mosby, St. Louis, 1982, p 2.

13. PETERSON, GH AND MEHL, LE: *Studies of psychological outcomes for various childbirth alternatives.* In STEWART, D AND STEWARD, L (EDS): *21st Century Obstetrics Now!* Vol. 1. NAPSAC, Inc., Marble Hill, Mo., 1978, p 210.

14. PETERSON, GH AND MEHL, LE: *Studies of psychological outcomes for various childbirth alternatives.* In STEWART, D AND STEWART, L (EDS): *21st Century Obstetrics Now!* Vol. 1. NAPSAC, Inc., Marble Hill, Mo., 1978, p 210.

15. SIMKIN, P. AND REINKE, C: *Planning Your Baby's Birth.* The Pennypress, Seattle, 1980, p. 1.

BIBLIOGRAPHY

ELKINS, VH: *The Rights of the Pregnant Parent.* Two Continents, New York, 1978.

EPSTEIN, JL: *Setting up a viable home birth service run by GNM's, backed by doctors and hospitals.* In STEWART, D AND STEWART, L (EDS): *21st Century Obstetrics Now!* Vol. 2. NAPSAC, Inc., Marble Hill, Mo., 1978.

FELDMAN, S: *Choices in Childbirth*. Grosset & Dunlap, New York, 1980.

GIMBEL, J AND NOCON, JJ: *The physiological basis for the Leboyer approach to childbirth*. J Obstet Gynecol Neonatal Nurs 6(1):11, 1977.

HAIRE, D: *The pregnant patient's bill of rights*. In STEWART, D AND STEWART, L: *21st Century Obstetrics Now!* Vol. 1. NAPSAC, Inc., Marble Hill, Mo., 1978.

HATHAWAY, M AND HATHAWAY, J: *Children at Birth*. Academy Publications, Sherman Oaks, Ca., 1978.

HOLMES, HB, ET AL (EDS): *Birth Control and Controlling Birth*. The HUMANA Press, Clifton, N.J., 1980.

L'ESPERANCE, CM: *Home birth—A manifestation of agression?* J Obstet Gynecol Neonatal Nurs 8(4):227, 1979.

LEBOYER, F: *Birth Without Violence*. Alfred A. Knopf, New York, 1978.

MATHER, S: *Women's interest in alternative maternity facilities*. J Nurse-Midwifery, 25(3):3, 1980.

MCKAY, SR: *Second stage labor—Has tradition replaced safety?* Am J Nurs 81:1016, 1981.

NOBLE, E: *Essential Exercises for the Childbearing Year*. Houghton Mifflin, Boston, 1976.

PARMA, S: *A family centered event? Preparing the child for sharing in the experience of childbirth*. J Nurse-Midwifery 24(3):5, 1979.

ROBERTS, J: *Alternative positions for childbirth. Part II: Second stage of labor*. J Nurse-Midwifery 25(5):13, 1980.

SUMMER, PE AND PHILLIPS, CR: *Birthing Rooms: Concept and Reality*. CV Mosby, St. Louis, 1981.

WOODS, NF: *Alternatives in childbirth*. In FOGEL, CI AND WOODS, NF: *Health Care of Women: A Nursing Perspective*. CV Mosby, St. Louis, 1981.

YOUCHA, G AND YOUCHA, S: *Where should baby be born? A guide to today's options in childbirth*. Woman's Day, April, 1981.

POST-TEST

1. The traditional setting for birth is _____ . Three nontraditional settings for birth are: (a) _____ , (b) _____ , and (c) _____ .

2. Complete the following table by using the key: A = always, U = usually, NU = not usually, S = seldom

	Hospital	Birthing Room	Birth Center	Home
parental control				
obstetric intervention				
parental choice of several birth companions				

	Hospital	Birthing Room	Birth Center	Home
prolonged contact with newborn				
personnel & equipment for complications				

3. Using the list below, identify five conditions that necessitate care in the traditional hospital setting:

   _____ clear amniotic fluid
   _____ 36 weeks gestation at onset of labor
   _____ ruptured membranes for 36 hours
   _____ estimated fetal weight of 7 lbs.
   _____ breech presentation
   _____ unmarried woman
   _____ hemoglobin of 8
   _____ blood pressure of 180/110

4. Complete column B by listing one alternative to the early labor routine described in column A.

Column A	Column B
Separation during admission	
Perineal shave	
Enema	
Bed rest	

5. List one advantage and one disadvantage to having friends or family, including children, present at birth.

	Advantages	Disadvantages
Friends/family		
Children		

6. Mrs. B. plans to have her 3- and 5-year-old children present at the birth of their new sibling. List four actions she should take to help make this a positive experience.

   a. _____
   b. _____
   c. _____
   d. _____

7. For the past two hours Mrs. M. has been sitting with the head of the bed elevated 45 degrees and with pillows under her knees and arms. She is comfortable, but her contractions do not seem to be increasing in frequency or intensity. Describe three other positions you can assist Mrs. M. to assume.

   a. _____
   b. _____
   c. _____

8. List two advantages and two disadvantages of electronic fetal monitoring.
   Advantages:
   a. _____
   b. _____
   Disadvantages:
   a. _____
   b. _____

9. For the past hour Mrs. M. has been lying on her back, lifting her shoulders up, and pulling her legs back and apart for pushing during her second stage contractions. The fetal head is not yet visible at the introitus.

   A. Describe three positions you can assist Mrs. M. to assume for pushing.
      1. _____
      2. _____
      3. _____

   B. What instructions can you give Mrs. M. for more effective pushing? _____
   _____
   _____

10. What measures can be taken to minimize the need for an episiotomy?
    a. During pregnancy: _____
    _____
    b. During delivery: _____
    _____

11. Using the list below, indicate which actions would facilitate parent-infant attachment.
    _____ placing the baby on the mother's abdomen immediately after birth
    _____ initial breastfeeding 8 hours after birth
    _____ separating mother and baby for recovery
    _____ administering silver nitrate eye drops immediately after delivery
    _____ father or mother cutting the cord
    _____ father holding the baby in the first hour after birth

Answers

1. The traditional setting for birth is the hospital; nontraditional settings are the birthing room, in- and out-of-hospital birth center, and the home.

2. Key: A = always, U = usually, NU = not usually, S = seldom

	Hospital	Birthing Room	Birth Center	Home
parental control	NU	U	A	A
obstetric intervention	U	NU	S	S
parental choice of several birth companions	S	U	A	A
prolonged contact with newborn	S	U	A	A
personnel & equipment for complications	A	A	U	NU

3. Of those conditions listed, the following necessitate care in the traditional hospital setting:
   36 weeks gestation at onset of labor
   ruptured membranes for 36 hours
   breech presentation
   hemoglobin of 8
   blood pressure of 180/110

4.

Early Labor Routines	Alternatives
Separation during admission	Give the partner the choice of staying with the woman or waiting in a lounge.
Perineal shave	Not shaving; clipping at home or in hospital.
Enema	No enema or small enema at home or in hospital.
Bed rest	Walking; lounging on couch, rocking chair, and so forth; visiting, playing cards, watching TV.

5.

Birth Companions	Advantages	Disadvantages
Friends/family	More relaxed atmosphere	Pressure to perform.
Children	Less sibling rivalry and regression. Shared family experience.	May misinterpret expressions of pain. May interfere.

6. The following measures should be taken to help make the presence of children at birth a positive experience:
   a. prepare the children for what to expect.
   b. let them know what they can and cannot do.
   c. have a support person for the children.
   d. allow them freedom to come and go at will.

e. acquaint them with the birth place beforehand (if other than the home).
7. Alternative positions for labor are:
   a. standing, walking around the room, leaning against her partner for support during contractions
   b. kneeling, resting her arms on the bed or chair for support
   c. side-lying in bed with the head of the bed elevated at least 30 degrees
   d. sitting in a chair or in bed with legs dangling over the side.
8. Advantages of electronic fetal monitoring:
   a. decreased stillbirths.
   b. decreased mental retardation.
   c. decreased cerebral palsy.
Disadvantages of electronic fetal monitoring:
   a. improved fetal outcome not consistently demonstrated by research.
   b. limitation of mobility.
   c. early and artificial rupture of membranes necessary.
   d. potential increase in maternal anxiety.
   e. increased cesarean delivery rate.
   f. with internal EFM, some increased postpartum endometritis and occasional newborn scalp abscesses.
9. a. Alternative positions for pushing are:
     1. side-lying, holding her bent upper leg up during contraction
     2. on her hands and knees
     3. sitting on the toilet or in bed with the head elevated more than 45 degrees, with her legs bent, relaxed, and apart
     4. squatting: (a) supported by her partner under the arms, (b) by a chair, or (c) in bed on a birthing stool
   b. Instructions to give for effective pushing are:
     1. push only when she has the urge
     2. contract only her abdominal muscles, keep rest of body, especially face, thighs, and pelvic floor, relaxed
     3. inhale, hold her breath, and push for as long and as hard as she feels the urge to
     4. keep her abdominal muscles contracted as she inhales between pushes
10. To minimize the need for an episiotomy, the following measures can be taken:
During pregnancy: perineal massage with oil
During delivery: position other than lithotomy; manual support of the perineum with warm compresses; pant to control the urge to push; ease the head out at the end of or between contractions

11. Of the actions listed, the following facilitate parent-infant attachment:
placing the baby on the mother's abdomen immediately after birth;
father or mother cutting the cord;
father holding the baby during the first hour after birth.

INDEX

A *t* following a page number indicates a table; an italic page number indicates an illustration.

Bradley method of, 226–227
breathing during, 224
eclectic approaches to, 231
hypnosis and, 227
Kitzinger method of, 229–230
Lamaze method of, 228–229, 232–245
breathing during, 233–234
techniques for, 239–241
concentration during, 233
positioning during, 233
methods of, 226–231
neuromuscular control and, 232
psychosexual method of, 229–230
reactions to labor and, 224
Read method of, 226
relaxation during labor and, 224
tension and, 234–235
Wright method of, 230
tension during, 234
exercises for, 234–235
Chloroprocaine, 195
Codeine, 188
Concentration
in Lamaze childbirth, 233
Contractions, uterine. *See* Uterine contractions (UC).
Creatinine
fetal maturity and, 154

DECELERATION
fetal heart rate and, 73–74, *74*, 75
Delivery
cesarean
inhalation anesthesia and, 209, 210
emergency, 35–37
nursing care during, 17–39
of placenta, 31
pain relief during
drugs for, 179–222
premature
nursing measures for, 159–160
vital signs following, 31
Delivery room
vs. labor room, 278–279
Demerol, 188–189
Descent

fetal, 16
promotion of, 99
of fetal head, 92
Diabetes
maternal
labor induction and, 139
Diagonal conjugate (DC), 92
Doppler unit, 63
Doptone, 63
Drug(s)
analgesics, 188–189
narcotic antagonists and, 189–190
beta-mimetic
premature labor and, 156
oxytocic
following delivery of placenta, 31
for labor induction, 141
sedative-hypnotics, 190–191
tocolytic
premature labor and, 156–159
use of
factors determining, 185–186
side effects of, 185–186, 188–193
supportive nursing measures with, 187
Dystocia
uterine, 61

ECLAMPSIA
labor induction and, 139
Effleurage, 237
Electronic fetal monitor(ing) (EFM), 66, *67*
continuous, 67–70
external, 68–69, *68*
internal, 69–70, *69*
oxytocin challenge test and, 78–79
Elimination
during labor, 25
Endometrium, 54, *54*
Enema(s)
as labor stimulant, 132–133
contraindications to, 132–133
during labor, 265
Engagement
fetal, 4
Epidural block